The Mary Kay Guide to Beauty

The Mary Kay Guide to Beauty

A Personal Guide to Looking and Feeling Your Best

The Beauty Experts
at Mary Kay Cosmetics

Addison-Wesley Publishing Company, Inc.

Reading, Massachusetts   Menlo Park, California
Don Mills, Ontario   Wokingham, England   Amsterdam   Bonn
Sydney   Singapore   Tokyo   Madrid   Bogotá
Santiago   San Juan

BCDEFGHIJ-KR-8987
Second Printing, July 1987

Writing	Susan Duff Elaine Raffel
Design and Layout	Jennie R. Bush of Designworks, Inc.
Photography and Illustration Direction	John Lemberg Elaine Raffel
Photography	Tim Boole, Steve Seeger, and Neill Whitlock
Styling	Jan Keeton Deborah Points
Makeup/Hair Styling	Gigi Coker Felini Cindy Gregg
Illustration	Phil French

The Mary Kay Guide to Beauty was set in ITC Garamond and Vivaldi by DEKR Corporation of Woburn, Massachusetts. International Colour Services, Inc., of Rochester, New York, supplied the separations and camera work. The book was printed on 70-pound Warrenflo paper from Lindenmeyr Paper Company of Boston, Massachusetts, at W. A. Krueger Company of New Berlin, Wisconsin.

Additional photo credits appear on page 240.

It is with great love, pride, and respect that we dedicate this book to all the beauty experts at Mary Kay Cosmetics — the independent beauty consultants who make up our organization. These remarkable women do so much more than teach skin care and makeup artistry. Each day they bring beauty into the lives of others, cheerfully giving of their time, knowledge, and experience.

Our beauty consultants are the reason Mary Kay Cosmetics has achieved so much in its first twenty years. Through their future efforts, millions of women (and maybe even a few men) will learn more about "beauty" in all its wonderful dimensions!

Foreword

Of all the lessons I've learned in the cosmetics business, one of the most universal is that women like to be told that they're beautiful. And why not? There's no nicer compliment. It's only natural that we feel better about ourselves when others offer their praise, support, and approval.

But did you ever stop to consider that the better you like yourself, the more beautiful you appear? It's a perpetual cycle: once you begin feeling your best — and believing that you are — you'll project that image to the world!

At Mary Kay Cosmetics, our goal has always been to help women bring the beauty they have inside them — outside! Instead of concentrating on what's less than perfect, we encourage them to look at the big picture — the positive qualities that make them special and unique. I don't know how many times I've heard a woman worry about her close-set eyes when she should have been focusing on their gorgeous shade of blue! It's not just coincidence that when you look past your shortcomings, others do too.

Still, that doesn't mean you can "wish" your way to an attractive appearance. Looking good takes motivation and effort. It means setting aside time to do those things that will contribute to your physical and your emotional well-being. Rule Number One: Include yourself on your list of priorities — no matter how long that list may be.

Believe me, I know how busy a typical day can be. There's your career, your family, your home, and dozens of other obligations. But stop and think how much better things seem to go on days when your energy level is high and you're feeling good about yourself. Somehow knowing you're in optimum form generates an unmistakable confidence, an attitude *and* assurance that can carry you through anything.

As for finding the time to devote to a sensible beauty routine, one of my favorite expressions is: You can do it! Just as work expands to fill the time available for it, you'll also be able to fit self-care and self-awareness into your daily life if you really want to. The key is not to think of this time as just an indulgence. Instead, consider it an important part of your life, necessary to keep you functioning in peak condition.

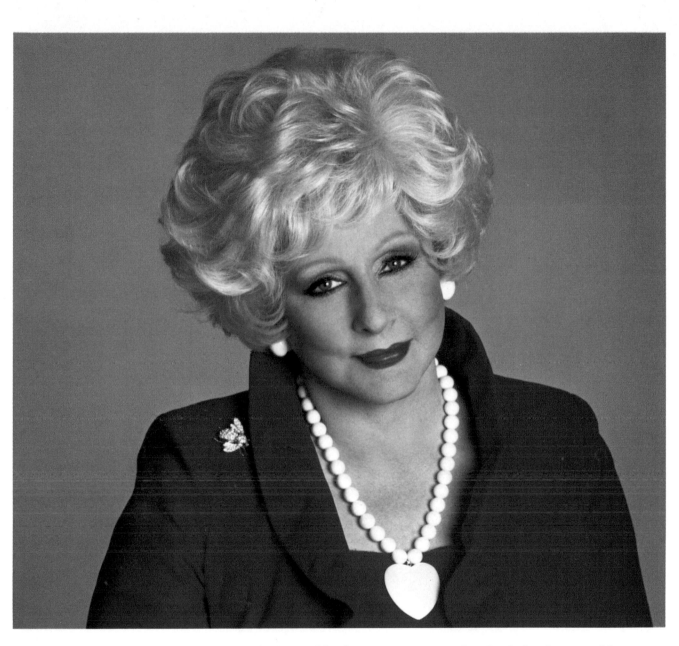

Yet inevitably there are women who think they're too old or too ugly or too unsuccessful ever to be beautiful. How wrong they are! Many's the time I've convinced a woman who felt that way just to try skin-care and beauty products. So often the results are magical. All of a sudden, that woman feels pretty — and it shows inside and out. From that point on, she becomes dedicated to her daily beauty routine.

This, of course, doesn't mean hours of fussing and primping. Nobody has that much time. Instead, I recommend a positive attitude and sense of self, discovering, step by step, exactly what makes *you* so special — and so beautiful.

Foreword

There's that word again — *beautiful*. Don't let it scare you. There's no need, since today's definition is so different from what it used to be. Beauty now is both accessible and attainable, including such qualities as energy, health, and vitality, radiance, confidence, and personal style.

So how do you reach your beauty potential? First, you need an intelligent plan of action with challenging, but always realistic, goals. We at Mary Kay Cosmetics believe everyone can climb the ladder of success, provided she moves up one rung at a time. And once you understand that this pertains to all aspects of your life — from skin care to diet to career — you'll be able to reach new heights.

I also encourage you to experiment, to grow, learn, and keep pace with what's going on in fashion, makeup, your field, and your world. When you step outside your comfort zone, I know you'll find the results to be well worth the effort.

Still another necessary element of being your best is believing in yourself — capitalizing on your assets and making the most of your talents. Then decide what changes you want to make and what areas you'd most like to improve. Once you know what it takes to make you feel terrific — and believe it's possible — you can start a positive move in that direction.

Finally, be sure you take advantage of what the experts have to offer. Whatever you need — information, encouragement, motivation, advice — don't hesitate to turn to those who have the knowledge and experience to guide you.

This book was designed to be a working tool — a source for direction, facts, and inspiration. As you read it, bear in mind that beauty is individual and personal, that the look and feeling you're after is one with which you can be happy and comfortable each and every day of your life.

The first step is the hardest: making a commitment to yourself, *for* yourself. But once you do it, you're well on your way!

Mary Kay

ontents

Your Special Beauty

Reflect on the real beauty within you that radiates to everyone you see. Your personal appeal begins with your view of yourself, the pleasure and joy you take in being who you are. Take a fresh, new look at yourself right now. Get to know and appreciate that special person. Then learn how to tap your inner beauty to create a personal style. Your beauty potential lies within.

Beauty Means...

You can always tell when a woman feels beautiful. She has an extra bounce in her stride, a gleam in her eyes, and a sparkle in her smile. Even if you can't pinpoint the exact cause, a woman who feels beautiful has an aura that comes from within: a special confidence and charisma people can't help but notice. That's why a single set of beauty standards doesn't work anymore. Today, women are free to develop their own style, to set their own goals and priorities, to make the choices and changes that affect their lives. Most important of all, they have the freedom to fulfill their potential — to take control of both their looks and their lives.

Personal beauty evolves from the interest you take in yourself. It comes from having commitment, energy, and a sincere desire to be your best. Whether you're a student, a homemaker, a career woman, or a grandmother, you have to start by making space in your life for beauty: reserving time for yourself — not as a bonus or a special indulgence, but as a regular, important part of your daily routine. Whatever your lifestyle, you can set up an ongoing self-care regimen that suits your individual needs. The key is education — taking an intelligent, positive, and realistic approach to beauty. It means understanding how your body functions; why skin and hair care are so essential; and how to use cosmetics for maximum benefit.

The Mary Kay Guide to Beauty addresses these issues — and many others. It provides you with the information you want to complement your own motivation and the knowledge you need to bring about effective, long-lasting results. In addition, we ask you some eye-opening questions designed to help you take a closer look and see yourself in a new, and perhaps different, light. These inventories should spark your imagination and expand your outlook. They should help you evaluate what you like best about yourself and help you envision and realize your most important beauty goals.

Beauty is not so much hard work as it is a commitment and a willingness to invest in yourself. We think you'll find that a regular beauty routine is one of the surest investments you'll ever make — because you're responsible for the returns. In the following pages, we introduce you to an approach to beauty that is easy, enjoyable, and flexible enough for even the busiest schedules. The best part is the dividends are tremendous. You'll feel happier, more alive, and more attractive. And as a result, you *will* be!

Knowing who you are and how special you can be means taking an interest in yourself — learning everything you can about your personal style of beauty, from the inside out. It's a fresh new outlook that starts here and lasts a lifetime, a philosophy of self-care that helps you make the most of your own good looks.

Important Basics

Every effective beauty plan should revolve around four important basics: skin care, glamour makeup, hair care, and a healthy, fit body. Together these elements contribute to your total look — which means each needs your special attention.

As you begin a routine, it may help to remember that beauty is an ongoing commitment for every woman. It calls for an active approach, based on positive, realistic actions and changes. You want it to be fun and exciting — something you look forward to. It shouldn't be complicated, time-consuming, or monotonous. The key is to look at the rewards: the luxury of devoting time to yourself, the confidence that goes hand in hand with looking your best, and the sheer pleasure of seeing the tangible benefits of your efforts.

There's no better feeling than knowing you're in peak condition. The more you learn, the more you want to learn. The more you accomplish, the higher you set your goals. You begin to welcome the responsibility of taking care of yourself — and, as a result, all your other responsibilities seem simpler and can be accomplished more smoothly.

Healthy, glowing **skin** is an essential part of any beauty look. Because your skin is unique, it takes more than mysterious lotions and creams to keep it looking radiant. It takes knowledge and a skin-care program based on products that work together to meet your special needs. In addition, you want to take full advantage of all the latest advances in scientific research and technology. In *The Mary Kay Guide to Beauty* we present five steps to beautiful skin: cleanse, stimulate, freshen, moisturize, and protect. By following this regimen and using the right products for your skin type, you can keep your complexion looking clear, fresh, and vibrant.

Next in your beauty routine is **glamour**. There's a wonderful feeling that naturally goes along with finding just the right makeup look and cosmetics. It could be a smoky, rich eye shadow, a sensational lip color, or a blush that gives you a sun-kissed glow. Glamour makeup can accentuate your best features. It also lets you enhance, define, color, and update your own special look. And with proper guidance, you can learn to camouflage and correct. Included in our glamour makeup section are tips and ideas for selecting cosmetics, as well as step-by-step instructions for creating the looks you desire to attain. In addition, you'll see how cosmetics can change the way

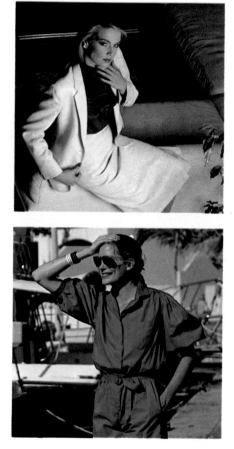

At work and at play, your beauty routine can make all the difference — clean, radiant skin; makeup that suits the occasion, your mood, and your unique style; shining, healthy hair; and a fit, toned body. The end result: a more beautiful you, every day.

When you put all the beauty basics together, the effect is naturally glowing — and yours alone. You've created your personal style by doing the most for yourself.

you feel about yourself — giving an important lift to both your appearance and your confidence.

Nothing enhances your glamorous image quite the way a flattering *hair* style can. For hair that is at its healthy best — clean, shiny, and manageable — you need a total, systematic approach to hair care. As with skin care, scientific developments have provided information to help you meet the individual needs of your hair type, whether it's dry, normal, or oily. Our hair-care section includes information on determining your hair type, along with guidelines for selecting the routine and hair-care products best suited to you. You'll find suggestions on style, cut, and color — which, with the advice of your hair stylist, will help you choose a look compatible with your hair type, face shape, personality, and lifestyle.

Finally, so many qualities of today's beauty look rely on a *body* that's toned, fit, and healthy. In addition to a basic program that shows you how to care for the skin all over your body, we show you how to get in shape with up-to-date information on exercise, relaxation, and all-around fitness. We also provide you with timeless, versatile wardrobe guidelines that will help you put together a look that is uniquely — and stylishly — yours.

The Mary Kay Guide to Beauty challenges you to develop your own personal beauty by instructing and inspiring you to become your very best. Use it as a guide to discover something new and beautiful about the way you look — and the way you *can* look.

Taking a Closer Look

Nothing does more for your appearance than feeling terrific. When you feel terrific, you possess a radiant glow and a healthy vitality. It's the way you look when something wonderful happens — when you're able to help someone, when you achieve a special goal, or when you're around those you love. Your inner beauty can't help but shine through.

Being beautiful becomes a total experience, a combination of the physical, the emotional, and the psychological. Many factors come into play — from the sparkle in your eyes to your easy, natural smile; from your genuine laugh to your graceful walk and confident posture. These features distinguish total beauty from just a pretty face. They help every woman look and feel her beautiful best.

The most effective beauty plans start from the inside. Like most clichés, "Beauty is more than skin deep" is true. It can be most beneficial to take time to think about your inner strengths — the many qualities that make you beautiful from within. You'll be better equipped to evaluate what you like most about yourself and what you might like to improve. The following inventory can help you start making these decisions. It was designed to put things in perspective, to help you honestly assess areas for change and growth, and to guide you in setting realistic goals and objectives.

Today, being beautiful calls for action, not perfection. The key is knowing what's important to you — what you want out of life — and accepting the challenge to become the best person you can be.

Vitality comes from within and gives your look that extra sparkle. Who you are shows beautifully in the way you look and the way others see you.

Read the statements below when you have time to relax and give them your complete attention. Look at yourself objectively and try not to think about how others might evaluate you. Circle those statements you feel best describe your strong points. Circle as many, or as few, as you like. Then turn to pages 18 and 19. Remember, this isn't a test, and no one can fail!

1. I'm good at helping people around me feel comfortable.
2. I have respect for who I am and what I do.
3. I don't compare myself to others, and I enjoy being me.
4. I feel sure of myself when I'm with others.
5. I feel that I'm a loving person who enjoys getting close to people.
6. I'm loyal to my friends, and I can be there for them if they need me.
7. My feelings toward my family members are warm, supportive, and understanding.
8. I enjoy the opposite sex and am comfortable in their company.
9. I like to give 100 percent of myself to projects I consider important.
10. I can rely on my personal or religious beliefs for courage when I need it.

11. When the going gets tough, I can keep going.
12. I'm able to recover from disappointments.
13. I set realistic goals and fulfill them.
14. I can determine what's most important to me and give those things my best attention.
15. I don't have to rely on others to start up new projects.
16. I'm open to other opinions, but I have confidence in my own ideas.
17. I'm capable of getting things done in cooperation with others.
18. I have my own interests outside my family and/or work.
19. I'm curious about the world around me, and I try to stay well informed.
20. I take an interest in some form of artistic expression that reflects my own, or another, culture.
21. I try to appreciate people who are quite different from me and learn from them.
22. I strive for my own personal success.
23. I use my time well, balancing my work responsibilities with personal interests.
24. I find the time and energy for the things I really want to do, both for myself and for others.
25. I laugh easily, and I like to make others laugh.
26. Even in bad times, I can laugh at myself.

27. I would describe myself as a giving and sympathetic person.
28. I enjoy sharing.
29. I feel confident that I can shape my own world and create a good future for myself.
30. I adjust to situations that aren't exactly what I'm used to.
31. I handle surprises, good or bad, well.
32. It's easy for me to feel excited about interesting new places, people, and projects.
33. When I feel something is wrong, I do my best to try to correct it.
34. Whatever my religious convictions, I have faith in the potential for good in humanity and in the world.
35. I don't expect my life to be perfect, but I tend to concentrate on what's good in it.
36. I feel positive about where my life is going.
37. I like the way I look, and I'm interested in exploring new ways of being attractive.

Discovering Yourself

Everyone has individual strengths and weaknesses. But by getting to know yourself better you can determine where you want to make changes. You can also establish ambitions, goals, and routines that coincide with your capabilities and lifestyle.

Because the way you see yourself and the way you look are inseparable, your special traits are reflected in your appearance and your image. The inventory statements have been grouped below to relate to several specific character traits that affect the outward expression of your inner personality. See which ones reflect your current strengths — and which ones are traits you'd like to work on.

Statements 1, 2, 3, and 4 relate to your **self-confidence** — your poise and ease with others, as well as your pride in yourself. If you circled any of these statements, your self-confidence is probably expressed in your facial expression and body movement. Self-confidence gives you a special radiance that shines in your eyes and imparts an added sense of self-esteem to your appearance.

If you identified with numbers 5 through 8, you have a high capacity for **intimacy**, and you are a good friend, an excellent family member, and popular in social gatherings. The inner quality of intimacy shows through in the way you look at people and speak to them. You maintain eye contact with people you're talking to, and you let your looks express your true nature so that people can get close to you.

If you found items 9 through 12 to be true, you rate high on **inner strength** and are more capable than most of seeing projects through. High energy and stamina are the virtues of people who have strength, and these qualities add an aura of power to the way you look.

Statements 13 through 17 relate to your sense of **direction**. If you circled these statements, it means you know how to set priorities and goals *and* fulfill them. You're independent and secure, and you like taking the initiative. Well-directed people radiate assurance and self-awareness; having a purposeful attitude toward your life can give your posture an extra lift and your entire physical appearance a genuine, straightforward beauty.

Numbers 18 through 21 relate to your **versatility**, showing that you're a person who is interested in the world around you, that you are outgoing and knowledgeable. Your versatility adds sparkle to

The real beauty of friendship is that it's ageless and timeless. Nothing makes you shine the way genuine loving and caring for others can.

Your many expressions and moods — pensive, happy, loving — show you're comfortable being yourself. A positive, healthy self-image is an essential beauty asset, a number-one priority for looking your radiant best.

your looks because your sincere interest in people, places, and things endows your beauty with the lively glow of an active mind.

Sentences 22 through 24 are about your *self-fulfillment*, your interest in success, and your ability to achieve. Your capacity to fulfill yourself as much as possible adds the quality of serene confidence to the way you look and gives your appearance its special note of self-assurance.

The last thirteen statements, numbers 25 through 37, relate to your *attitude* — how you feel about yourself, your life, and the world around you. If you thought these ideas expressed your view of life, you are positive, optimistic, and enthusiastic — all high-energy qualities that give your looks extra impact. Your attitude is also reflected in your generosity, flexibility, and ability to adapt when necessary, as it is in your charity and sense of humor. These characteristics show up in the way you treat yourself and others.

Inner beauty is where total beauty begins. If you feel good about yourself, you'll look better, too. Read on. You'll find lots of ideas for making your inner beauty work for you — today and for the rest of your life.

BEAUTY MEANS...
Self-Confidence

Self-confidence is a quality that's *essential* to how attractive you are and how attractive you feel.

Self-confidence comes from knowing, and liking, who you are. It allows you to be yourself, to hold your own in everything you do.

Having confidence in yourself shows in your poised self-assurance — the way you have of making everyone around you feel good (because *you* feel so good!). It comes from taking pride in yourself and what you do. Self-confidence is simply self-esteem — appreciating yourself and *showing it!*

One of the best ways to boost your self-confidence is to learn how to enjoy yourself. That means more than having a good time with others. It means concentrating on what's best about you, and taking on the challenge of accomplishing what you want to change about yourself.

Self-confidence also means self-respect — respect for your body, your mind, and your spirit. That comes from taking good care of yourself. Staying healthy so your body functions well. Staying alert to the world around you to keep your mind in shape. Staying true to yourself to keep your spirit wholesome. Respecting who you are sometimes means standing up for your beliefs and ideas — and learning how to do it gracefully.

Self-confidence comes from your ability to concentrate on yourself — not in a selfish, narcissistic way, but in a way that allows you to be aware of both your gifts and your shortcomings. If you think positively about your own strengths, you aren't tempted to measure yourself against someone else. There will always be someone who can outdo you at something. Having self-confidence means recognizing that no one else is quite like you, and that it is therefore pointless to compare yourself to others. It doesn't mean being blind to your faults. It means being in touch with your best inner self. It means trusting yourself, and believing that you can be the kind of person you want to be.

You take on new challenges and expect the best because you *know* you can do it. Your faith in yourself gives you energy, strength, verve — the confidence you need to create your individual style of beauty.

Self-confidence is your key to personal success. You believe in yourself and trust your abilities. You understand and appreciate your unique qualities. There's no one else quite like you.

Intimacy

The ability to get close, to understand and listen, to love — that's what intimacy is. Your personal warmth gives you a glow that embraces everyone around you and makes them feel as good as you do.

Intimacy is that special capacity you have for getting close to people, for getting involved in what's important.

Intimacy is personal warmth; it comes from your ability to open up and let others know exactly who you are. Intimacy is sharing yourself — giving your all to your family and friends, getting close to the people who are meaningful in your life. And, of course, it can mean falling in love.

Intimacy means having the courage to get involved . . . with the special people you love, and with the rest of your world. Your ability to be intimate comes from your attitude toward people in general. When you understand your own needs, you are open to responding to human needs all around you. You can give everything you do that little bit extra because you want to, and because getting close to people is important to you.

You can develop your capacity for intimacy simply by being a warm and caring friend, by being an understanding parent and family member, by looking for ways to make all your relationships closer and more meaningful, Sometimes it means a gesture — a phone call to a sick friend or a present for a special birthday. Often, though, it simply means being a good listener and having a good heart. You'll find opportunities to develop intimacy every day if you look for them.

People who are capable of intimacy are people we love. We trust them with our feelings because they have trusted us with theirs. We can tell them our problems and know they'll try to understand. We can laugh easily with them because we know they take sincere pleasure in our joy. We can even cry with them because we know they are not afraid of their own emotions, or of ours.

Intimacy means not being afraid of who you are, and wanting to share yourself with the people you love. It means being able to love — and be loved.

Inner Strength

Inner strength is your faith in yourself and your own abilities, the power you have within you to make good things happen and to bounce back when disappointments come.

Inner strength is a kind of internal energy; it can come from your relationships, from your religion, or from your commitment to make the most of who you are. It gives you the potential to strive for excellence and achieve it, to hold on to your convictions and apply them to everything you do, to be strong for others as well as for yourself.

Sometimes, it's easier to *appear* to be strong than it is to really *be* strong within. No matter what the circumstances, inner strength is derived from what you possess internally: your faith in yourself, the responsibility you feel toward the people who love you, your standards and beliefs — your character.

Inner strength comes from having learned how to deal with mistakes, misunderstandings, and even bad luck. It means learning how to work out whatever may go wrong — from a stalled car to a major family crisis.

When you're strong internally, you can count on yourself and others can count on you, too. You take responsibility for yourself and know how to shoulder your own burdens. And, when the people who are important to you need your help, they know they can rely on you.

Having inner strength means being a self-starter, a person who can initiate difficult new projects without the help of others. Inner strength also gives you the emotional wisdom and the internal energy to start again when those projects sometimes fail.

Inner strength is the power you have inside you to cope with the worst as well as the best; to take on the world with optimism whatever it brings; to take risks without fear of failure; and to accept failure by learning from it.

Your capacity to share — to pass on to family and friends what you know and love — gives special meaning to your life. Others know they can rely on you because you know you can rely on yourself.

Inner strength gives your life direction. It means being a self-starter and having the initiative, energy, and determination to accomplish your goals and fulfill your needs.

Versatility

Because of your versatility, you not only are open to new ideas — you enjoy the unfamiliar and the unexpected. You take the time to cultivate your interests and are able to meet new challenges with confidence.

You take advantage of every opportunity to learn, and you find new experiences appealing. You appreciate insights others share; they help you see your world in a new and different light.

Versatility means taking an interest in your world and exploring its many facets, finding what fascinates you and developing your own special talents.

Versatility is an expansive outlook on everything around you, the ability to go beyond your life's boundaries to discover new interests. It comes from cultivating an appreciation of people, places, and ideas that are different or unfamiliar to you, and it gives you the desire to learn as much as you can from every situation, and to expand your life beyond its everyday horizons.

Versatility means acquiring an adventurous perspective on being alive; reaching out to embrace the new; excelling in a variety of personal skills; being curious and informed; viewing the universe as a bountiful source of wonder in which you want to be involved.

Being versatile means developing more than one dimension of yourself — not locking yourself into any one role or mold, and not limiting yourself to rigid restrictions imposed on you by others or by yourself.

You can develop versatility by expanding your own expectations of yourself, by going beyond what you know you can do well to discover new and challenging areas of yourself. You become versatile when you take the time to cultivate your own potential interests. Whether it involves learning to knit an afghan or accepting a job promotion, versatility helps you meet challenges with confidence.

Being versatile will also make you feel better about yourself. Absorbing new information and being curious about the world will make you more interesting, more animated. You'll find you have more to say to people — at home, at parties, or on the job. Reading the newspaper every day, attending classes at the Y, or simply teaching yourself a new skill are all part of versatility.

When you're versatile, you are open to all that's new and exciting. You appreciate people who are different from you because you know you can learn from them. You're capable of adapting to the unfamiliar and you're comfortable with yourself in almost any situation.

Versatility offers you an introduction to as many situations, places, and people as you find interesting; it gives you the ability to play as hard as you work, and to discover the very best in yourself and your world.

Direction

Having direction is setting your own goals and striving for them, knowing what your priorities are and giving them primary attention. It's taking the initiative getting projects started, moving toward what you want, and feeling secure about where you want to go.

Having direction is approaching your life with the sound conviction that your aims are realistic and achievable. It comes from your ability to concentrate on what's important and to dedicate your energy to your most meaningful goals. It's having a sense of purpose.

Having direction means taking the straightforward path toward your destinations, being sure of where you're headed because you know your goals are right for you. And sometimes it means taking a less traveled, more difficult road because it's the only one that can take you to exactly where you want to be. A strong sense of direction can help you be a better friend and parent. Sometimes we use direction for personal goals — to start a new career or lose weight, for example. It takes a lot of energy to do either, and a good sense of inner direction can help you channel that energy to achieve the best results. Living your life with a sense of direction involves having a strong sense of who you are and what you want.

You can put direction into your life by defining your most important goals: the areas in which you want to excel, the milestones you're confident you can attain. Do you want to go back to school? Be a more patient listener? Climb the corporate ladder? Direction is what keeps you moving forward.

Direction gives you the ability to shape your own future. It gives purpose and an overall design to your everyday activities. Direction gives you a perspective on almost everything you do, and helps you understand how to get where you want to go.

When you have a clear sense of direction, you are willing to consider the many different roads that can lead to your destination. You are willing to be patient while determining the very best course for realizing your ambitions.

Believing in your dreams and planning ways to make them come true gives you direction. So does taking yourself and your goals seriously. Having direction means paying attention to what really matters to you and disregarding unimportant distractions. It means having confidence in yourself and your abilities.

You strive for what you want because your goals are important to you and you know you can achieve them. Your sense of direction adds structure and meaning to your life; it gives you purpose and strength, the determination you need to get what you want.

The beauty of giving your all to make your dreams come true is that fantasies *can* become reality; you'll find that your highest aims are within your grasp when you're willing to reach for them.

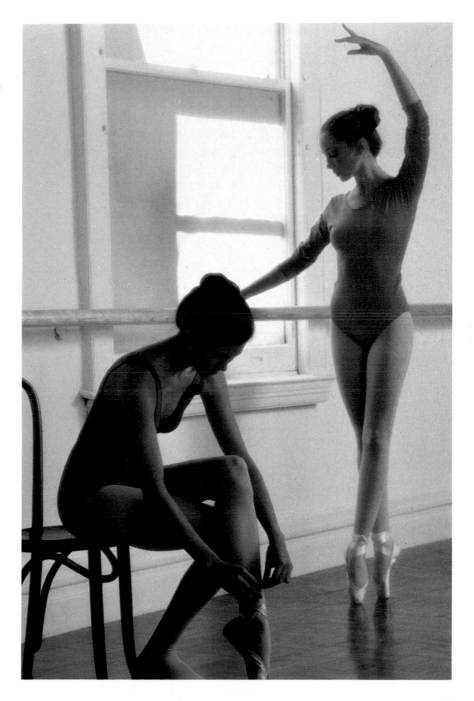

Self-Fulfillment

Self-fulfillment is your commitment to achievement in every area of your life. It's an ability to devote everything you have to doing your best and your sense of balance in deciding what success means to you — both personally and in your work life.

Self-fulfillment is what your goals are based on, the reason you strive to achieve them. It's understanding yourself, your needs and desires, and how you can best accomplish them. It's orienting your world toward attaining your own personal satisfaction, as well as being aware of the fulfillment you can derive from others.

Self-fulfillment means having a healthy awareness that only you can really make yourself happy. Fulfilling yourself begins with understanding what makes you feel best about yourself and your life. It comes from knowing who you are in relation to the world around you. It helps you make the right decisions, based on your own self-knowledge.

Self-fulfillment means developing a clear sense of what's really rewarding to you — not only the outward appearances of success, but emotional gratification as well. It also means putting all the elements of your life — work, family, and friends — into a balanced perspective. You have to know what makes you feel best. You could be as fulfilled by a simple, private activity that's meaningful to you as by receiving public acclaim. Fulfillment is very personal, and specifically related to what you alone want from life. Sometimes it involves compromise, trading off a career for children, or a promotion for a job you like better.

Being self-fulfilled gives you a spirit of generosity: when you know what makes you feel good, you want to share it with others, and you want to help them fulfill themselves.

Self-fulfillment requires energy and commitment. What really fulfills you may not be easily attainable, or the challenge itself may offer you the most fulfillment. Fulfilling yourself isn't always easy, but it's always worth the effort.

You treasure those moments that give you so much happiness — simple pleasures that reward and enrich your life. Self-fulfillment comes from the smallest task done well or from a challenging project finally completed. It's a feeling of satisfaction that comes from achieving what you set out to do.

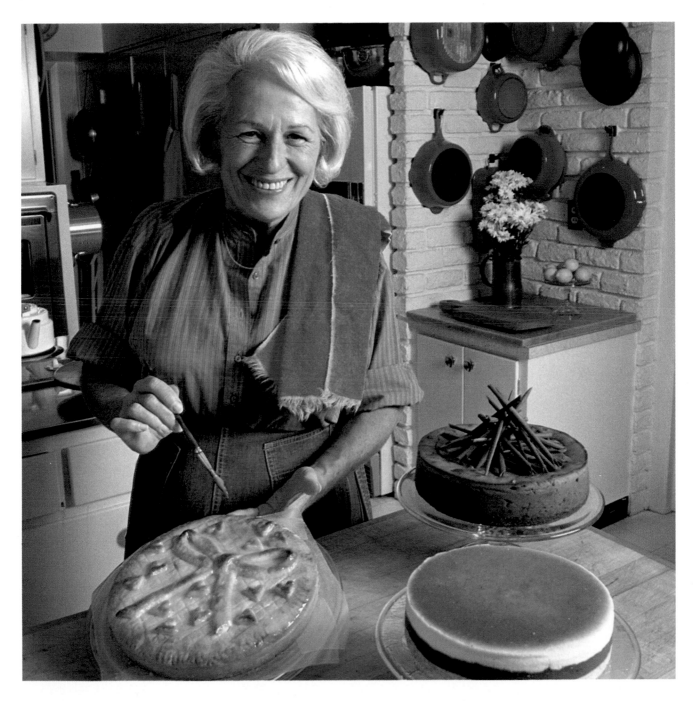

A Positive Attitude

A positive attitude is represented by your positive perspective on yourself and all of life around you, your enthusiasm for what excites you, and your optimism for the kind of future you know you can create. It's your compassion and generosity, your ability to change when change is for the good, and a sense of humor that becomes your saving grace in the worst of times.

Attitude is the source of your whole personality — the way you see the world and the way the world sees you. When you have a healthy, positive attitude you know how to apply constructive intelligence to your problems as well as your goals; your self-assurance allows you to enjoy being you; your fine-tuned self-awareness both perceives and expresses what you know to be right and good.

A positive attitude means having an outgoing involvement in yourself and the people you care about, a day-by-day joy in making the most of whatever life brings you — not complaining about what life fails to bring you. A positive attitude comes from your personal enthusiasm, your wholehearted zest for the life and people you love.

Being positive means looking for the potential in even the worst situations. It's approaching each day knowing that everything can't always be perfect, but believing that there is good to be found almost everywhere, and knowing you have the ability to try to change what you feel is wrong.

Optimism is the source of a positive attitude, and optimism comes from your own intelligent perspective on your capacity to make things better. When you believe in your own self-worth, you also believe in discovering what is worthwhile in everyone around you, and you look for the best in others.

A positive attitude gives you sincere enthusiasm for what really excites you, and allows you to become exuberantly involved in all your interests. It makes you the kind of person who can give others the strength and confidence to persevere in the worst of times, and even to laugh when everything goes wrong.

Having a positive attitude means finding joy and delight wherever they exist, and discovering them in unlikely places. The sources of a positive attitude are faith in humanity's potential for good and a sound belief in your own possibilities for excellence.

Your positive attitude makes others glad to be around you; your optimism is contagious. You feel good about your world because you feel so good about yourself — and that makes others feel good, too. There's always a bright side, and you know how to find it.

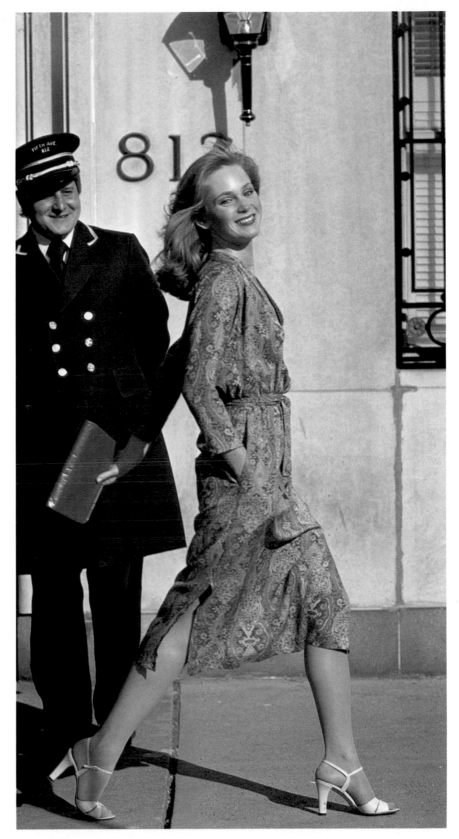

Your enthusiasm, energy, and confidence show through in everything you do. Others can't help noticing that something special about you when you look and feel your best.

33

Looking Good

Your special beauty is yours alone. It comes from not only knowing but liking who you are. The time, thought, and energy you invest in understanding and enhancing yourself are worth the effort; the reward is that you bring the beauty you feel inside, outside.

Looking good — it means presenting the most attractive person you are capable of being to the world around you and taking an interest in your appearance. It's putting energy into what you look like and making yourself glow with all the qualities of inner beauty you know you possess.

Looking good is making the most of what is uniquely yours — not comparing yourself to others, but rejoicing in your own beauty. It's discovering the special allure that belongs to you alone — and making the *very most of it.*

Looking good means consistently doing what is best for you, establishing the best beauty habits and taking care of yourself because you know it matters: because you know *you* matter, and you want the world to know it too!

Looking good is letting your inner beauty radiate outward, presenting yourself to the world as a woman who knows what's beautiful about herself.

Looking good is paying attention to your appearance because you know it's important, and because it's so closely related to the way you feel about yourself. It's taking the time to express who you are in the way you look.

Good looks come from taking the time to understand the effect your appearance has on the people you deal with every day, from putting energy into adopting the right beauty habits. What fun it is to have someone cast an admiring eye on you, or smile when you walk into a room. Looking good is realizing your potential for being at your best in every sense.

Looking good starts with taking good care of yourself, learning as much as you can about making the most of how you appear to others. It's projecting the best of who you are onto the way you look every day. Whether getting ready to go to work or preparing for a special evening, you know how good it feels to look your best, and the way your inner feelings show up in your outward appearance makes all the difference.

Looking good is feeling good about who you are and glowing with your own special beauty.

Making It Yours

How do you take advantage of your special beauty? By putting your energy and caring into a presentation of yourself that radiates what's most beautiful from within. It shows on the outside in the polish and sparkle that come from taking the best possible care of your appearance.

Making it yours is using all your resources to make the most of yourself. It's creating a balance between who you are inwardly and how good you look outwardly. It's taking all the elements of your inner beauty and letting them shine through, adding a special sparkle to your eyes, projecting energy into your stride, giving a warm, healthy glow to your skin and a special graceful charm to your expression.

Making it yours means knowing what you have, understanding your potential, and taking an interest in developing it fully. Making it yours is what this book is about — taking the most advanced, effective, and efficient beauty techniques available and making them as much a part of you as your most beautiful inner qualities.

Your *self-confidence*: the special quality of knowing and liking yourself, an element of who you are that shows up beautifully in every expression and movement. Your capacity for *intimacy*: the personal warmth that adds a very special glow to the way you look. Your *inner strength*: the sense of wholesome energy that gives your looks dynamic power. Your *versatility*: the extra sparkle you get from having many facets to your personality. Your sense of *direction*: the positive motivation that animates your person. Your *self-fulfillment*: the way your contentment with yourself gives you an extra aura of beauty. Your *positive attitude*: the expression of your prettiest feature, your smile. *Looking good*: your ability to find what's best about who you are and let it show beautifully.

Skin Care

Total beauty begins with beautiful skin that is clean, fresh, and glowing. Your skin reflects the special care and knowledge you invest in your health, your state of mind, and your appearance. Well-cared-for skin is the basis of your overall beauty plan and your personal style. It's time to make successful skin care a goal — to learn how to achieve and maintain a soft, smooth, and radiant complexion.

Your Skin

Beauty may begin within, but a personalized skin-care program can enhance your physical beauty. To make any skin-care program work for you, you must understand the nature of your skin: what it is; how it functions; why it looks and feels as it does.

Few people realize that skin is the largest organ of the body. Through it you experience the sense of touch and feel temperature, texture, and pressure. Your skin, a sensitive organ, is vital to your entire physiological system; it helps to keep your body temperature normal, which in turn keeps your internal organs functioning as they should. Your skin protects your body from harmful foreign substances, harmful bacteria, and some of the damaging ultraviolet rays from the sun. It also helps retain essential body fluids and heals most of its own wounds.

Your skin has a highly specialized two-layer structure that is constantly regenerating itself. The upper layer of skin you see — the *stratum corneum* — is composed of flat, dead skin cells that contain the protein *keratin*. Beneath these dead skin cells is a layer of living cells. Together they form the skin's outermost layer, the *epidermis*. In healthy skin, new cells are generated in the lower level of the epidermis and move to the surface. The top older cells harden, die, and are then shed from the surface steadily in microscopic flakes. This whole process is continually repeated in a four-week cycle.

The upper layer of the epidermis acts as a barrier to prevent the entry of harmful bacteria into the lower, more vulnerable levels of skin, where infections can occur. This layer also slows the rate of moisture loss from lower layers of the skin. Harsh soaps or detergents can irritate skin by removing oils from the surface of the skin and damaging the protective barrier.

Beneath this paper-thin epidermis is a layer of skin, fifteen to forty times thicker than the epidermis, called the *dermis*. The dermis is composed of collagen and elastin fibers that support the vital components of the skin — the blood vessels, nerves, sweat glands, hair follicles, and sebaceous (oil) glands. *Fibrocytes*, cells that produce the collagen fibers, are also found in the dermis.

Many blood vessels and capillaries supply nutrients and oxygen to the skin. These *blood vessels* also help keep body temperature at a healthy level by contracting and expanding in response to external

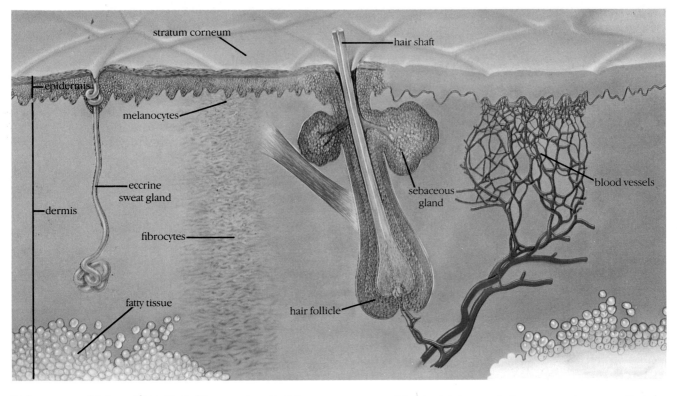

Labels on the illustration:
- stratum corneum
- hair shaft
- epidermis
- melanocytes
- eccrine sweat gland
- sebaceous gland
- blood vessels
- dermis
- fibrocytes
- fatty tissue
- hair follicle

Below your skin's surface is an intricate system composed of many parts.

stimuli. When you arc suddenly frightened, for example, your facial skin blanches. The blood vessels in your dermis contract, directing the blood (which helps supply color to your face) away from your skin and toward your body's tensed muscles. On the other hand, when you become overly warm from exertion, the blood vessels in your dermis expand so that heat from the center of your body moves to the outside, normalizing body temperature. In the process, skin tends to redden.

The most common sweat glands, the *eccrine glands*, also help control body temperature. These glands look like small coiled tubes that extend up through the epidermis and open onto the surface of the skin as pores. Sweat glands constantly bring small amounts of water (mixed with salt and waste products such as urea) to the surface of the skin. When the weather is very hot, or when your body becomes very warm, greater amounts of water are transported to the sweat pores, where the perspiration evaporates and cools the surface of your skin to prevent your body from overheating.

Hair grows in *hair follicles*, tubes located throughout the dermal layer of the skin, although the follicles are really extensions of the epidermis. On animals, hair serves a protective function. On man, hair on the head protects the scalp from sunburn, while eyelashes and eyebrows shield eyes from foreign substances. (Eyelashes, like the hair on your scalp, are shed and replaced regularly. Occasional loss of lashes should not be cause for alarm.)

Your Skin

The *sebaceous glands* — the source of the skin's natural oil supply — are attached to the hair follicles. They produce an oily substance called sebum, which they secrete into the follicles and onto the hair shafts for distribution over the skin's surface. Sebum coats the outermost layer of the skin, and is thought to help keep skin soft and pliable.

The sebum, in combination with surface moisture, forms a coating on the top layer of skin. Normally at an acidic pH level, this coating may help prevent bacterial infections and contribute to the protective barrier function of the epidermis. The moisture and oil supply on the skin's surface is constantly replenished. Because of the skin's "buffering capacity," or ability to adjust its own pH, cosmetic and skin-care products with a pH balance slightly different from that of the skin do not usually disturb its natural protective coating for a significant period of time.

At the lower levels of the epidermis, and to some extent at the very top of the dermal layer, *melanocytes* — cells containing the pigment melanin — give skin its color. The size of melanin granules produced by the cells and the amount of melanin within them determine the shade — light, medium, or dark — and/or consistency of the skin's pigmentation. Skin color is principally hereditary, but the melanocytes can be influenced by several factors over time, such as pregnancy or exposure to the sun. Freckles are concentrations of melanin that occur in small patches.

Below the dermis, a layer of fatty tissue gives the skin its shape and insulates the body against extreme temperature changes, absorbs some physical trauma, and serves as a reservoir of energy. There is generally very little of this fatty tissue under facial skin; most of what's there is located in the chin and cheek areas.

Also underlying the dermis are muscles that connect it to the bones of the skull. We use muscles to form various facial expressions — smiling, frowning, and squinting. Some of the muscles perform involuntary movements, such as blinking. (Even when our faces are relatively still, the small muscles underlying the facial surface remain somewhat tense to hold the shape of the face.)

The facial surface does not retain the contours and lines of every expression because of elasticity — a property of the collagen and elastin fibers in the dermis. Elasticity is also affected by water in the

Whether you're awake or asleep, your skin performs its functions twenty-four hours a day. Proper skin care is vital to the health and appearance of your skin.

Healthy skin is essential to looking good. The more you know about what your skin is and what it does, the better you can make it look and feel.

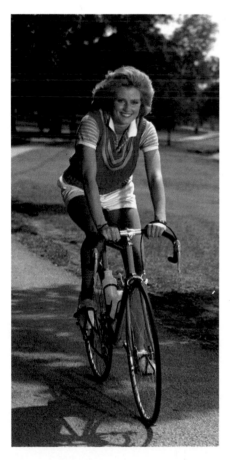

epidermis. Dry skin, which may be insufficiently supplied with moisture and oil, may therefore retain these small expression lines more easily than other skin types. Facial expressions are one of the principal causes (along with exposure to the sun) of the deeper wrinkling of the skin.

The goal of proper skin care, as outlined in the pages to come, is to keep your skin functioning at peak performance, to make it look and feel soft, smooth, and beautiful. A good skin-care routine can supplement the natural processes that keep your skin healthy and vibrant. The result: a naturally beautiful you!

Special Considerations

Skin is a highly responsive organ. It reacts to the internal changes in your body, as well as to the environment around you. The condition of your skin can change in response to some of these internal and external considerations, so it is sometimes necessary to modify your normal skin-care routine to accommodate such factors as age, hormonal influences, and environment.

Age The most significant change in your skin as you grow older occurs in the dermis. The sebaceous glands may become less active and produce less oil. Poorly lubricated skin may not retain water as easily, and as a result, your facial surface may dry out. You should remember to use foundations and moisturizers more frequently to prevent your skin from looking and feeling tight. If your skin has been oily throughout your lifetime, the visible effects of aging will be minimized. If your skin has always been dry, the dehydration that accompanies aging will be more damaging.

Your skin also becomes less elastic with age. The lines you form when you move your face may become deeper and more noticeable. Additionally, the collagen and elastin fibers in the dermis become less effective in supporting the skin and keeping it elastic. These natural processes of aging cause the skin to wrinkle and lose its firm texture. Exposure to sunlight accelerates the wrinkling process. Using a sunscreen under your makeup becomes even more important, therefore, as you age.

The goal of a good skin-care program is to minimize the effects of aging on your skin. You can't turn back the clock, but you can take steps to protect your skin against external factors.

You're never too young — or too old — to practice a program of daily skin care. By taking good care of your skin you can help minimize the effects of aging.

Hormonal Influences Starting at puberty, changing hormone levels contribute to the hyperactivity of the oil glands and may lead to the formation of acne. During your adult life, hormonal levels may also fluctuate to a greater or lesser degree, usually in correspondence with your menstrual cycle and pregnancy.

Various hormones are released throughout your twenty-eight-day menstrual cycle. Some of these hormones stimulate the oil glands, which produce a greater amount of sebum just prior to a menstrual period (and often during and following menstruation). The greater amount of oil production can sometimes be associated with pimples and breakouts (see pages 48 and 49). In addition, research indicates that certain oral contraceptives (particularly the mini-pill and those containing high amounts of synthetic progestins called androgen-dominant pills) contribute to oiliness of the skin and acne formation. These situations can call for a change in your skin-care routine at different points in your menstrual cycle. Using a mask and freshener more frequently may be helpful in controlling excess oil on the skin (see pages 60 to 63).

If your skin is dry, you may be less apt to be affected by hormonal fluctuations during the menstrual cycle. Even dry skin, however, may break out before and during menstruation. If this occurs, you may want to reduce your use of moisturizer and/or night cream during that part of your cycle.

Pregnancy also changes the hormone levels in your body. Your skin may become either very dry and sensitive or excessively oily during pregnancy. If your skin becomes dry, increase your use of moisturizer and night cream. If your skin becomes oily, use a facial mask and freshener more frequently than usual, and reduce your usage of night cream or moisturizer.

Hormonal changes during pregnancy may also increase the production of melanin in your skin, which can result in a number of usually temporary pigmentary disorders, such as freckles and discoloration of certain skin areas. Dark patches, known as chloasma or mask of pregnancy, sometimes appear on the cheeks, near the mouth, or in the brow area during pregnancy. Irregular pigmentation increases with exposure to the sun; it is recommended that all pregnant women use a highly protective sunscreen (SPF 10 to 15) whenever they are going to be in sunlight.

Special Considerations

The top layer of your skin, the epidermis, is your body's single largest and most effective protector from damaging environmental substances. It prevents many toxic materials from getting through your skin's surface and minimizes water loss from deeper tissues. Cleansing removes environmental pollution or soils from the *surface* of your skin, making it look, feel, and function better.

The coating of oil from the sebaceous glands and water from the eccrine sweat glands increases the protective function of the epidermis. In areas where the climate is extremely dry, this coating evaporates so rapidly that it becomes difficult for the oil glands to replenish lubricants on the facial surface. The use of protective cosmetics — foundations and/or moisturizers — helps hold the important water content of the skin's surface.

To conserve body heat when the weather is very cold, the blood vessels in the dermis constrict. It is a good idea to keep your face, neck, and ears well covered in winter, to help keep your skin warm. When skin is warm, the blood vessels can more easily supply necessary nutrients to the skin. In cold weather, too, moisturizer can help protect against moisture loss.

In very hot weather, the sebaceous and sweat glands become more active, supplying extra oil and water to the skin's surface. In hot, dry climates, much of this excess water evaporates naturally. In hot, humid conditions, large amounts of oil can accumulate on the skin, and acne breakouts may be more frequent (see page 49).

The sun is the environmental factor that is most harmful to the health and appearance of your skin. Ultraviolet radiation — the element of sunlight that most seriously affects the skin — can cause permanent damage if you allow it to penetrate your skin. Ultraviolet rays deteriorate the dermis's collagen and elastin fibers, which provide your skin with its elasticity and ability to resist permanent wrinkling. Sun exposure breaks down these substances; the result is skin that sags, loses elasticity, wrinkles, and forms creases. The effects are cumulative. Increasing evidence also links severe sunburn early in life to serious forms of skin cancer later on.

Exposure to the sun does have some benefits. Sun exposure increases the available blood volume that circulates throughout the body, giving us a sense of well-being. It also provides us with vitamin

For maximum effectiveness, apply a sunscreen seven to fifteen minutes before your skin will be exposed to the sun.

Choose a sunscreen product you can spread evenly in a thick film on your facial skin; thin and uneven applications do not provide sufficient protection.

Apply sunscreen to all the exposed areas of your head, including the part in your hair, the tops of your ears, the top of your brow, your neck, and your neckline. Another sensitive area to remember is the tops of your feet if you wear sandals or go barefoot.

Protection is important no matter how dark your skin is. Even very tan or black skin is vulnerable to ultraviolet radiation.

If you engage in sports that make you perspire, reapply sunscreen regularly to maintain its effectiveness.

Ultraviolet radiation penetrates water, so use your sunscreen when you swim, and reapply it afterward.

Ultraviolet rays penetrate clouds and haze, so use a sunscreen even when the sun isn't shining. And don't feel an umbrella at the beach is sufficient protection. Sand can reflect rays, so you should wear a sunscreen anytime you're at the beach.

Sun damage occurs whenever you are in the sun, not just when you are most conscious of it. Time spent outdoors shopping, gardening, or walking can add up to more sun exposure over a lifetime than time spent at the beach, by a pool, biking, swimming, or boating. Always protect your skin with a sunscreen when you know you will be outdoors.

D for our bones, teeth, and hormonal systems. But weigh the advantages against the disadvantages of sun exposure, and consider that its benefits still exist when you apply a sunscreen. The use of a sunscreen to maintain a smooth and youthful complexion is perhaps the most important element in caring for your skin. A sunscreen with a sun protection factor (SPF) of at least 10 blocks most of the sun's ultraviolet radiation before it can damage your skin. (The SPF number indicates the length of time a given product will protect your skin. Using a sunscreen with an SPF of 10, a person who begins to burn within twenty minutes of exposure to bright noonday sun can tolerate the same kind of sun ten times longer, or almost four hours, before burning.)

Your heredity and the amount of time you spend in the sun can compound the risks and make the use of a sunscreen even more important in protecting the health and appearance of your skin. The danger of sun damage increases if you are fair-haired and/or fair-skinned, or freckle easily; if you live in the Sun Belt; or if your occupation or leisure activities keep you regularly exposed to strong sun. Other significant factors include:

Time of year: exposure to ultraviolet rays reaches its dangerous peak on June 21 in the northern hemisphere, lasting through August; but you need protection as early as April, long before the hottest days of August.

Time of day: the sun's rays are most intense, and thus most dangerous, between 10:00 A.M. and 2:00 P.M. (11:00 A.M. and 3:00 P.M. daylight saving time).

Altitude: at high altitudes, where the atmosphere is thinner, more ultraviolet radiation reaches your skin. You need protection whether you're working or vacationing in mountain regions.

Latitude: the closer you travel to the equator, the greater the amount of ultraviolet radiation. Exposure to ultraviolet radiation — and its concomitant risks — is twice as great in Dallas as in Chicago, for example.

Cumulative and permanent damage from sun exposure can be avoided by using an effective sunscreen. Keep the tips at left in mind. And make protection a natural part of your health-and-beauty-care regimen. It takes just a few minutes, and you'll be glad you didn't neglect it.

Special Considerations

Many of the milder problems you may encounter on your facial skin are caused by extremes in skin type — overly dry or overly oily, for example — and can often be improved with proper skin care. Some problems, however, require specialized care or professional treatment.

Allergies tend to be different in different people. Your way of life — what you eat, where you live, prescription drugs you take — can increase or diminish your allergies. If you notice an allergic reaction — a rash and/or swelling of the skin — and suspect any cleansing or cosmetic product you use on your skin, stop using the product immediately. Take its list of ingredients to a dermatologist or allergist who can help you identify which ingredient is causing the problem and suggest possible alternative products for you to use.

If you use cosmetic preparations *in combination* and develop an allergic response, try a ruling-out procedure. Use no cosmetics at all and observe your skin for one to five days. If the allergic reaction improves dramatically or disappears within this period, you may assume that it was associated with one of the products you used. Next, use a small amount of one product at a time for a minimum of five days, carefully observing your skin's reaction to it. If a reaction occurs, discontinue using that product. When you discover which product caused the allergy, seek a dermatologist's or allergist's aid if you wish to be patch-tested for individual ingredients.

Two other common skin disorders are ***seborrheic dermatitis*** and ***rosacea***. The rash of seborrheic dermatitis is red and scaly, and most often occurs on the scalp, in the areas of the eyebrow, along the edges of the nose, and behind the ears. It can easily be mistaken for dryness, but unlike common dry skin, this condition does not improve when a moisturizer is used. Rosacea is a face rash that produces redness and pimples in adults, especially on the nose, mid-forehead, chin, and cheeks. Causes of the rash are unknown, but it has been found that in some cases the condition is aggravated by the ingestion of alcoholic beverages, spicy foods, coffee, or tea. A dermatologist can diagnose and treat these conditions.

Lack of melanin in a specific area of the skin may produce white patches, a condition called ***vitiligo***. Conversely, excessive pigmentation on certain parts of the skin surface produces dark areas; ***birthmarks*** are a form of hyperpigmentation. If such pigmentary

Surface irregularities on the skin begin below its surface. When the hair follicle fills with dead skin cells, bacteria, and oils, it can lead to an open comedo, or blackhead, as illustrated here, or to a pimple. Good skin care can help prevent unsightly breakouts.

Acne: A Common Skin Condition

While acne is generally associated with puberty, this condition can also appear for the first time in adults in their twenties or thirties. At any age, heredity, drugs, or oily cosmetics can add excess oil to skin already oversupplied with sebum. Other causes may include comedogenic (pore-clogging) chemicals, stress, heat, and humidity.

Acne was once thought to be caused by certain foods or dirty skin. Today, acne is believed to be associated with overly oily skin and genetic and psychological factors, such as stress. The latest acne research reports that it is probably a result of a buildup of keratin proteins, bacteria, and oils in the ducts (exits) of some hair follicles; large follicles located on the face, chest, and upper back are most susceptible.

In teenagers, rapidly rising hormone levels cause the sebaceous (oil) glands to enlarge and produce more oil. These same hormones can cause excess keratin to plug follicle openings, resulting in the most basic type of acne lesion, the *comedo*.

Comedones are composed of bacteria trapped in the hair follicles together with dead skin cells and oil (sebum). Normally, skin cells shed while in the process of moving up to the skin's surface; comedones form when the cells aren't shed, filling up the follicles. Some comedones may develop into the typical inflamed acne lesions.

Pimples and pustules can develop from comedones when the walls of the plugged follicles rupture, spreading the dead skin cells, oil, and bacteria into the dermis. The blood vessels below the skin then become enlarged to accommodate more white blood cells, which are needed to combat the infection in the lower layers of the skin. The enlarged blood vessels cause the skin to appear red, and the white blood cells combine with the dead skin cells, sebum, and bacteria impacted in the follicle to form pus. The result is a red pimple with a yellowish head, called a pustule, which forms on the surface of the skin.

Once the pimple has formed, it is unwise to squeeze out the material trapped there; at worst, it forces bacteria deeper into the skin and can cause scarring.

If pustules form on your face, chest, and/or back, consult a dermatologist.

If your skin is prone to acne-type breakouts, keep it clean so that excess sebum, bacteria, and dead skin cells on the skin's surface do not contribute to pore blockage. However, once acne is present, excessive scrubbing or frequent cleansing will not control it, and any rough manipulation of the skin may further irritate and inflame the lesions. Diet is no longer considered to be significant as a cause of acne in most individuals. However, if you suspect a particular food as the cause of an occasional pimple, remove that food from your diet for a few weeks and observe your skin to see if its condition improves.

Medical research has developed a variety of ways to treat differing stages and degrees of acne. If you suspect you have incipient acne or the condition is apparent on your skin, consult a dermatologist as soon as possible.

disorders disturb you, seek medical advice.

Another common form of hyperpigmentation is *facial moles*. These usually harmless spots sometimes sprout hair. However, if you notice an obvious sudden change in a mole, or if one begins to bleed, consult a dermatologist immediately.

Cold sores and *fever blisters* are caused by a form of the herpes virus, for which there is currently no known cure. Vaccines are now being tested and may be available within a few years. The virus remains in the skin where it first erupted and can be aggravated to run its course again by sunburn, scratching, or stress.

Facial warts, which are also caused by a virus, can be removed. Your dermatologist can advise you concerning treatment.

$\mathcal{T}$aking a Closer Look

The type of skin you have determines how you should care for it. The following questionnaire will help you identify your apparent skin type and the kind of skin-care routine you should follow. Keep in mind that this inventory can give you only a very general classification of the condition of your skin. It may change with age as well as with the seasons. You are also likely to observe improvements once you've established a proper program for skin care.

Mark the boxes below that best describe the way your skin looks and feels at this point in your life. Then look at the skin type listed beneath the column in which you marked the most boxes; this is your skin type at this time. As your skin changes, you will want to take this inventory again; it's best to review your answers about four times a year, at the beginning of each season. Your answers may also depend on the type of products you have recently been using to care for your skin.

Magnified views (from left to right) of small, medium, and large pores.

---

1. Six hours after cleansing, my skin usually feels:

| ☐ Very dry to moderately dry | ☐ Relatively unchanged: well-lubricated but not oily or dry | ☐ Oily on my forehead, nose, and chin (the T-zone), drier on cheeks and sides of face | ☐ Very oily |

2. Three hours after applying a typical liquid foundation (one not formulated for any specific skin type), my facial surface appears:

| ☐ Matte (dull) in finish, with no shine | ☐ Soft and smooth, neither dull nor shiny | ☐ Somewhat shiny in my T-zone | ☐ Very shiny |

3. Whiteheads, blackheads, and small bumps appear on my facial skin:

| ☐ Almost never | ☐ Very rarely, possibly before and/or during menstruation | ☐ Sometimes, especially on my forehead or chin or near my nose | ☐ Almost always |

4. The small lines that form on my face with facial movements tend to remain "imprinted" on my skin:

| ☐ Around my mouth and eyes and on my forehead | ☐ Very faintly near my eyes, and increasingly as I get older | ☐ Just around my eyes, and possibly near my mouth | ☐ For a short time, then they disappear |

5. My facial pores are:

| ☐ So small they can barely be seen | ☐ Small to medium and regular in size over the surface of my whole face | ☐ Medium to large; noticeably larger in my T-zone | ☐ Large, especially in my T-zone and on my cheeks |

6. As compared to five years ago, my facial skin has become:

| ☐ Quite a bit drier | ☐ Slightly drier | ☐ Drier only on the sides of my cheeks and the outside edges of my face | ☐ Not noticeably drier; possibly more oily |

| DRY | NORMAL | COMBINATION | OILY |

50

7. Regardless of the products I use, my skin feels tight and dry:

☐ Often
☐ Occasionally in extremely cold or dry weather
☐ Only on the sides of my cheeks and the outside edges of my face
☐ Rarely or never

8. Some areas of my face tend to become oily:

☐ Rarely
☐ Occasionally, in extremely hot or humid weather
☐ Usually in my T-zone
☐ Almost always

9. My skin tends to chap:

☐ Frequently, on both my hands and face
☐ Occasionally, on both my hands and face, when exposed to extremely dry or cold weather
☐ Only on the sides of my cheeks and the outside edges of my face; possibly on my hands
☐ Rarely or never on my face; sometimes on my hands, in extremely dry or cold weather

DRY	NORMAL	COMBINATION	OILY

Your Skin Type

Record your skin type and the date you have taken this inventory in the space provided below. Look for special considerations for your skin type throughout this book to help establish the best skin-care and beauty program for yourself. If you change your diet, or you find yourself in a dramatically different climate, or you start or stop taking medication, review this inventory again a few weeks after such a change. Each time you take the inventory, note the changes and improvements in your skin so you can make appropriate adjustments in your beauty routine.

Date	Skin type	Remarks
_____	_____	_____
_____	_____	_____
_____	_____	_____
_____	_____	_____
_____	_____	_____

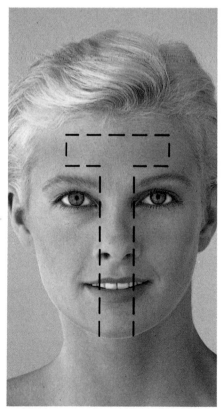

The T-zone

$\mathcal{D}$iscovering Your Skin Type

No one has skin exactly like anyone else. In order for your skin-care program to work effectively, your routine must be designed to meet the individual needs of *your* skin. There are basically four types of skin — dry, normal, combination, and oily. The personal inventory of skin type on pages 50 and 51 can help you determine which category describes your own skin.

Dry skin is usually characterized by small pores and a matte (dull) finish, with little or no superficial shine. Expression lines form readily on dry skin, first on the brow, then around the eyes and near the lips. Dry skin is most typical in women over the age of thirty-five and those who live in either hot or cold low-humidity climates. Dry skin may also develop among women who spend a great deal of time outdoors without properly protecting their skin from the elements. Such skin becomes rough and may flake or crack.

Because environmental factors dry the surface of your face without actually affecting the deeper sebaceous glands that produce and secrete your skin's oils, it is sometimes difficult to determine whether you really have dry skin. Our personal inventory of skin type helps you explore the nature of your skin in a way that will enable you to recognize your skin's true type and adjust your skin-care program accordingly.

Normal skin has a smooth texture and, at best, a fine, porcelain-like quality. Lines and wrinkles seldom form on this type of skin until rather late in life. Normal skin rarely, if ever, develops white-heads, blackheads, or pimples.

Although many women may describe their skin as normal, it is actually a rather rare type. If you are lucky enough to have been born with normal skin (for, in fact, heredity is a major factor behind skin type), you need a good program of care to maintain its excellent condition.

Combination skin is probably the most common skin type among women in their twenties and thirties. It is characterized by moderate to very oily conditions in the T-zone (the area forming a T across the forehead and down the center of the face, running down the nose and onto the chin), combined with variably dry skin at the outside edges of the face — cheeks, temples, outer corners of the eyes, jawline, and possibly the areas surrounding the upper lip and the corners of the mouth.

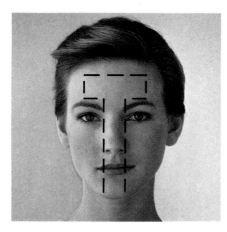

The T-zone

The appearance of combination skin varies from a shiny and large-pored texture in the T-zone to smaller pores and a more matte finish of the outer edges of the face. This type of skin can be cared for with a regular and healthful skin-care program that controls oil in oily areas and adds moisture to drier areas.

Oily skin results when the sebaceous glands produce too much oil, giving skin a shiny appearance, and sometimes a greasy or sticky feel. Oily skin tends to wrinkle less readily than drier skin types. The large amount of oil on the skin's surface may help the upper layers hold onto water and protects the skin from environmental causes of dryness. However, this skin type is prone to acne-type breakouts well beyond adolescence. Good skin care can help control excess oiliness and the formation of whiteheads, blackheads, and pimples. Oily skin usually has larger pores than other skin types. Use of the proper skin-care products and procedures helps make the pores appear smaller and the face smoother and less shiny.

Although you can't change your skin type, you can change the condition of your skin with proper care and adequate protection. After completing your personal inventory of skin type, you will be able to note special considerations and recommendations for your skin type throughout the five steps to beautiful skin, which follow. Knowing your skin type allows you to personalize your skin-care routine and to take that first step toward your own special beauty.

5 steps to *Beautiful Skin*

Your skin is the translucent background for your expressive features and for the glamorous makeup you apply. A careful program of skin care soon results in skin that is smooth, soft, and glowing — skin that displays the pride you take in yourself and your desire to look and feel your best. A clear, radiant complexion may sometimes seem hard to achieve, but it is attainable by everyone, and it is the first and most important step to a woman's total beauty.

The five steps to beautiful skin — cleanse, retexture, freshen, moisture balance, and protect — form a beauty-care program based on scientific research about what is best for your skin. Each of the steps has a scientific basis related to the many roles your skin plays every day. For your skin-care program to work effectively, it is important that you use all five steps. Each step is simple to perform, and together they can become a very pleasant and relaxing part of your daily beauty routine.

The five steps to beautiful skin work well for each of the four different skin types — dry, normal, combination, and oily. While no skin-care program can change your skin type, the five steps to beautiful skin can improve the condition of your skin and accentuate its most positive elements.

In the pages that follow, you will learn the scientific importance of each step, how to choose appropriate products for your specific skin type, and how and when to apply them. Everything you need and want to know about your personal skin-care program is right here at your fingertips. You'll soon want to make the five steps to beautiful skin a part of your daily beauty routine.

1 *Cleanse*
Creams and cleansers soften and smooth your skin while they gently and effectively remove makeup, surface oils, and impurities.

2 *Retexture*
A refreshing facial mask removes dry surface cells and stimulates circulation while improving and enhancing skin's texture.

54

3

4

5

3 *Freshen*
A freshener tones, softens, and conditions as it balances the pH of the skin's surface. Freshening further stimulates circulation and removes any residue of previous products.

4 *Moisture Balance*
Moisture balance products provide and hold in essential moisture as they minimize signs of aging. Dry areas feel softer, oily areas feel fresher. Moisture balancing products soften and condition your skin as they improve its resiliency and elasticity.

5 *Protect*
Foundation protects skin from environmental elements as it covers minor imperfections. It also provides a subtle hint of color to give skin a smooth, even-toned finish. Facial under-makeup sunscreen is also important in the protect step, guarding skin from the sun's damaging ultraviolet rays.

STEP 1

Cleanse

Your skin is exposed to many elements every day. Cleansing removes the substances that can accumulate on your face — makeup, excess oil (sebum), dirt and pollutants, and dead skin cells. These substances may contribute to pore-clogging and prevent the top layer of skin from functioning efficiently. For optimum results, choose a cleansing product that's non-comedogenic, fragrance free, and clinically tested for skin irritancy and allergy. Use the specific formula best suited to your individual skin type.

Dry skin tends to produce a minimal amount of natural oil and water for lubricating the skin, so a cleanser for this skin type must be able to remove both superficial impurities and dry, flaking skin cells *without* removing the necessary oil and moisture on the skin's surface. A rich, highly emollient cleansing cream is recommended for dry skin.

Normal and combination skins require the same cleansing treatment. It must loosen and remove cosmetics and surface soils, lift off dead skin cells, and clear away excess oil, particularly in the T-zone area of the face.

An effective cleanser for both these skin types should cleanse the face and pick up extra oils where they have accumulated; at the same time it shouldn't dry other, less oily parts of the face. A light, creamy cleanser is the best formula for these two skin types.

Oily skin requires special cleansing because the excess sebum that coats the facial surface may tend to trap dead skin cells. In addition, soils adhere more readily to oily skin and may be more difficult to remove. The best cleanser for oily skin is one that effectively loosens and removes surface soils, dead skin cells, and a larger amount of excess oil without stripping away the skin's natural moisture. A light, pearlized liquid cleanser that produces a sudsy lather with water is the best formula for oily skin.

Whatever your skin type, a daily cleansing routine is a must. It's also important to cleanse in the proper manner, using a special technique that we'll describe on pages 58 and 59.

City life can be tough on your skin; air pollution and other environmental soils may interfere with your skin's functions. A daily cleansing routine helps counteract the potential damage of an urban environment.

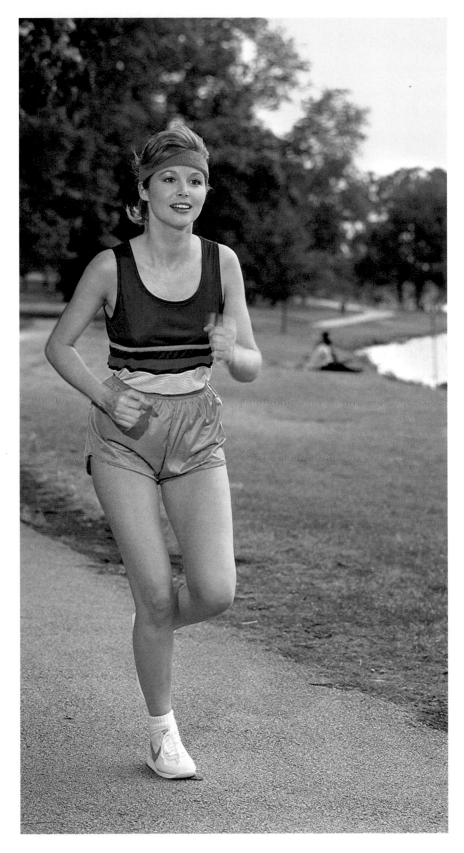

Glowing good looks are within
your reach — and they start with
an ongoing skin-care routine. Step
number one: cleansing, to help
keep skin clear and fresh.

Cleanse

When using any cleansing product, apply it gently to avoid pulling the delicate surface of your skin. Begin by putting the cleanser on your fingertips; then, starting at the base of your throat, lightly stroke upward and outward. Move upward over your chin, jawline, the area surrounding your mouth, nose, and on to the sides of your cheeks and temples. Next, work the cleanser upward and outward over your forehead, just above the eyebrows, and upward to the hairline. When you apply any product near your eyes, always use your ring finger to exert the least amount of pressure in this delicate area where facial skin is thinnest. Below your eyes, stroke gently inward from the outside of your eyes toward the bridge of your nose. Avoid scrubbing or harshly manipulating any area of your face — tugging or pulling skin can damage fragile tissues and promote wrinkling.

Dry, normal, and combination skins should be cleansed in the manner described above. Apply the cleansing product recommended for your skin type with light strokes of the fingers. A gentle massaging action will enhance the cleansing effect. Remove cleansing cream with a wet facial cloth; liquid cleanser with a wet facial cloth, or by rinsing with warm water.

Oily skin should be cleansed with a foaming product, which is applied somewhat differently. Work cleanser for this skin type into a lather by adding a small amount of water. Rinse off with warm water or remove with a wet facial cloth.

When to Cleanse All skin types should cleanse twice a day — in the morning, to soften, smooth, and remove excess oil that might have accumulated on the skin overnight; and in the evening, to remove the day's makeup, dirt, and oil. (Those with dry skin, however, may want to cleanse only once a day, in the evening, especially if the weather is cold and dry.) Always be sure to remove any residue of cleanser at the sides of your mouth, in the crevices near your nostrils, in the delicate eye area, and along your hairline and jawline. Regular cleansing will leave your complexion clear, fresh, and smooth — ready for the skin care steps to follow.

Movement of application: Always use an upward and outward motion to follow the natural orientation of your skin's dermal fibers. Never pull or tug, which can damage skin's delicate surface.

Cleansing feels great — and gives
your skin a healthy glow. For the
fresh feeling of properly cleansed
skin, apply the cleanser recommended for your skin type, using
the movement of application
shown at left. Next, dampen a face-
cloth with warm water and remove
the cleanser gently and thoroughly,
or rinse completely with warm
water. Make the most of this important step in your personal
beauty routine; you'll see and feel
the benefits. Cleansing is the first
essential step in your daily skin-
care routine.

Retexture

Because the cells on the top layer of your skin are continually being replaced, dead cells can accumulate and lead to a slowdown in normal epidermal functions. Regular use of a facial mask helps to remove these dry surface cells, exposing younger, newer skin. Pores appear more refined, circulation is stimulated, and impurities are removed, leaving skin fresher and brighter. Some masking products can also be used as a scrub for immediate sloughing of dry surface cells. Choose a mask that is non-comedogenic, fragrance free, and clinically tested for skin irritancy and allergy.

Dry and normal skins need a mask with a non-drying, moisturizing formula to remove dry surface cells and improve skin's elasticity. It should also have a creamy texture and contain natural oils and emollients to hydrate the skin and help make it soft and supple.

Combination and oily skins will benefit most from a clay-based formula, which contains oil-absorbing materials and a natural abrasive to exfoliate dead skin cells. It should thoroughly cleanse the skin, refine skin's texture, and help make pores appear smaller.

How and When to Retexture Masking products should be applied over the face using an upward and outward motion. Always avoid the eye and mouth areas. (Follow the movement pictured at the right.) As a mask, leave on for about ten minutes, then remove with a warm, damp facial cloth. If used as a scrub, massage lightly onto damp skin, again working upward and outward. Rinse with warm water or remove with a warm, damp facial cloth.

All skin types should mask twice a week at regular intervals, after cleansing and before freshening. If skin is very oily, or tends to be oilier in hot or humid conditions, you may want to mask more often — perhaps as frequently as every other day.

Proper movement of application

The stimulation of a mask does wonders for the condition of your skin. This second step is relaxing and beautifying; it leaves your skin feeling refreshed, vibrant, and alive. Apply the facial mask recommended for your skin type with featherlike strokes in the manner shown above; avoid the delicate areas around your eyes and mouth. After allowing the mask to dry (approximately ten minutes), or using it as a scrub, place a warm, wet facecloth over your mask to soften it for removal. Wipe off the mask gently, using the recommended movement of application. For best results, mask at least twice a week.

Freshen

Skin freshener does just what its name implies: it freshens the skin by completing the cleansing process and removing any residue of previous products. Fresheners also tone, condition, and balance the pH of the skin's surface as they further stimulate circulation, leaving skin softer and smoother. The product you choose should be formulated for your skin type, non-comedogenic, fragrance free, and clinically tested for skin irritancy and allergy.

Dry skin requires a gentle, alcohol-free freshener that will enhance the skin's natural ability to hold moisture. It should rehydrate your complexion and help wash away dry, flaky skin so skin looks fresher and more radiant.

Normal, combination, and oily skins will achieve best results with an alcohol-based freshener that equilibrates skin's oil balance. It should also help control oily buildup on the skin's surface and improve the texture of your complexion, so pores appear smaller and more refined.

How and When to Freshen Apply a few drops of freshener to a cotton pad and smooth over face and throat. Work in an upward and outward direction, using the movement of application illustrated at right. Repeat the process until the cotton shows no trace of dirt or makeup. Let dry naturally.

Always freshen twice a day, morning and evening — after cleansing or masking.

Proper movement of application

Luxuriate in the smoothness of skin freshened daily. This important step refines your pores, further stimulates circulation, and removes the residue of any previously used product. Moisten a cotton ball with a few drops of the freshener for your skin type. Apply it with gentle upward and outward strokes, avoiding the delicate areas around your eyes and mouth, as shown at right. Allow the freshener to dry naturally. Your skin will immediately look brighter, feel fresher.

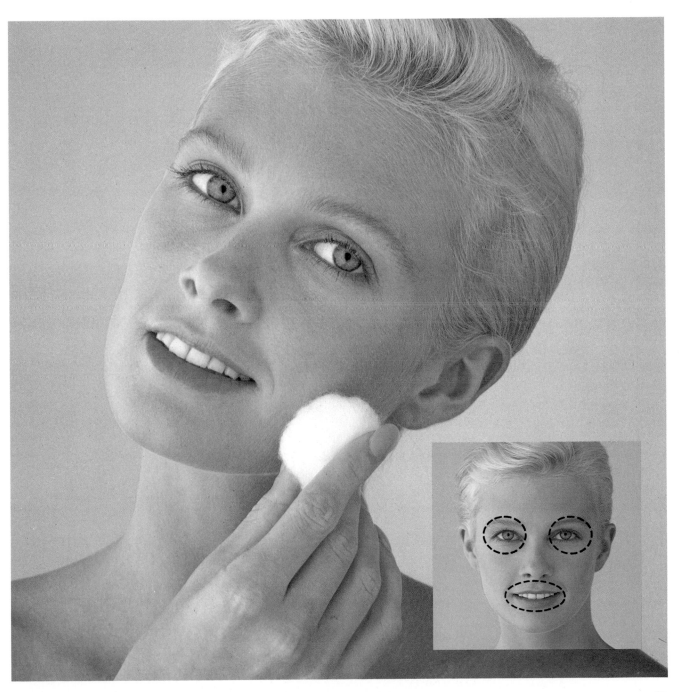

Moisture Balance

Moisture balance products are recommended for all skin types to help your complexion achieve and maintain its optimum moisture balance — neither dry nor oily. This step also softens and conditions skin, improves resiliency and elasticity, and provides a protective shield against environmental elements. Consistent use of a moisture balance product will help minimize the appearance of fine lines and wrinkles, so skin looks younger, smoother, and more vibrant. When selecting a moisture balance product, choose one that is non-comedogenic, fragrance free, and clinically tested for skin irritancy and allergy.

In addition to a lotion you use daily, you may also want to add a treatment cream to your skin-care regimen to provide extra moisturization when and where it's needed. This type of rich, emollient cream will help replenish essential intercellular lipids, reinforcing your skin's own moisture retention capabilities. In addition, a treatment cream will help control signs of aging as it improves the overall fitness of your complexion.

Dry skin, which loses water more rapidly than other types of skin, requires an emollient, enriched moisturizer day and night to minimize moisture evaporation. It will also relieve tightness and soften skin, providing a smoother surface for applying makeup.

Normal and combination skins need a fine-textured, skin-balancing moisturizer day and night to help skin maintain its optimum surface moisture level. Oily and dry areas are adjusted to a properly hydrated state so skin looks and feels soft and conditioned.

Oily skin will benefit from a lightweight, oil-controlling lotion that contains ingredients to absorb oil as well as to properly hydrate drier areas. This type of moisture balance product also helps makeup last longer, leaving a fresh, matte finish.

How and When to Moisture Balance Gently smooth your moisture balance product over your face and throat every morning and evening after freshening. Use light, feathery strokes, following the movement of application pictured at right. Those with very oily skin may want to apply a second coat of oil-controlling lotion for extra protection against oil breakthrough and shine.

Proper movement of application

When using a treatment cream, apply lightly with fingertips, again following the proper application movement. If you have drier skin, smooth on face and throat at night and under your regular moisture balance product during the day. Those with oilier skin should use this type of cream only on drier areas — around the eyes or on the throat. Treatment creams are especially beneficial during winter months to protect skin from the drying effects of cold and wind.

Consistent use of a moisture balance product suited to your skin type will help your complexion look its youngest and most vibrant. This step also helps your skin maintain its optimum moisture balance — dry areas are soft and conditioned, oily areas are smooth and fresh.

STEP 4
Moisture Balance

Your skin's moisture balancing needs may vary with changes in the seasons or with travel from one climate to another. Generally, heat causes your skin's oil glands to become more active. When weather is also humid, oil and water cannot evaporate naturally, so oils remain on the skin, coating the facial surface.

In hot and dry weather, the heat may stimulate excess oil production. But water tends to evaporate from the skin's surface in a dry atmosphere, so excessive oiliness is not such a great problem. Dry skin, however, can suffer in this climate because hot, dry air can lead to extreme dehydration. When exposed to the sun daily, your skin requires protection (see pages 46–47 and 73).

In cold and dry conditions, your oil production may become sluggish, limiting the supply of oil to your skin. Also, when the air is dry, water is lost rapidly from the skin's surface. These conditions can cause chapping, especially in cold, windy weather.

Humid air, which helps facial skin hold onto its moisture content, is beneficial to most skin types. However, cold and damp conditions can affect dry skin problems; hot and damp conditions can affect oily skin problems.

Both the cool, dry environment of air conditioning and the hot, dry conditions of artificial heating can dry your skin. In addition, since indoor cooling and heating systems counteract the outdoor climate, your skin may react erratically after being subjected to widely varying conditions. You must take all these changes into account when you use the chart at right. If you live in a hot, humid climate, but spend most of your time in an air-conditioned office and house, you should follow the moisturizing suggestions for a cold, dry environment. Similarly, if you live in a cold and damp area but are usually indoors in heated rooms, you should follow the suggestions for a hot, dry environment.

The chart offers guidelines on moisturizing your skin, but you should also use your own senses of sight and touch to note your skin's reactions. Whenever your skin feels greasier and looks shinier than usual, use your moisture balance product on dry areas only, or switch to an oil controlling formulation, and possibly use a mask more often. When your skin feels tight, change to a richer formula moisture balance product or use a treatment cream in addition to your regular skin care program.

Moisture Balance Needs in Different Climates

Skin Type	Environment			
	Hot and Humid	Cold and Dry	Hot and Dry	Cold and Damp
Dry	Use an enriched moisturizer under foundation during the day and alone at night. If extra moisturization is needed, use a rich treatment cream; if skin needs less moisturization, switch to a skin balancing moisturizer.	Use both a rich treatment cream and an enriched moisturizer under foundation during the day and alone at night.	Use an enriched moisturizer under foundation during the day and a rich treatment cream at night.	Use an enriched moisturizer under foundation during the day and alone at night. In cold, windy weather, also use a rich treatment cream.
Normal	Use a skin balancing moisturizer under foundation during the day and alone at night. Apply a rich treatment cream to dry areas.	Use a skin balancing moisturizer under foundation during the day. Apply a rich treatment cream at night and for extra moisturization under your regular daytime moisturizer when needed.	Use a skin balancing moisturizer under foundation during the day and alone at night. Apply a rich treatment cream to dry areas.	Use a skin balancing moisturizer under foundation during the day and alone at night. Apply a rich treatment cream to dry areas.
Combination	Use a skin balancing moisturizer under foundation during the day and alone at night.	Use a skin balancing moisturizer under foundation during the day and alone at night. Apply a rich treatment cream to dry areas only.	Use a skin balancing moisturizer under foundation during the day and alone at night. Apply a rich treatment cream to dry areas.	Use a skin balancing moisturizer under foundation during the day and alone at night. Apply a rich treatment cream to dry areas.
Oily	Use an oil controlling conditioner under foundation during the day and alone at night. Apply a second thin layer over the first for extra oil control.	Use an oil controlling conditioner under foundation during the day and alone at night. Apply a rich treatment cream to dry areas — around the eyes and throat.	Use an oil controlling conditioner under foundation during the day and alone at night. Apply a second thin layer over the first for extra oil control. Apply a rich treatment cream to any occasional dry areas — around the eyes and throat.	Use an oil controlling conditioner under foundation during the day and alone at night. Apply a rich treatment cream to dry areas — around the eyes and your throat.

Protect

The final step in your five steps to beautiful skin is the essential protect step — the application of foundation and, when needed, sunscreen. A foundation provides protection from environmental elements as it covers minor imperfections and gives your complexion a smooth, even-toned finish. The most beneficial formulas are non-comedogenic and clinically tested for skin irritancy and allergy. A sunscreen, worn under foundation, is also recommended to guard against the sun's damaging ultraviolet rays.

Dry and normal skins benefit from a creamy, oil-based foundation that helps provide and seal in moisture as it protects from dehydrating conditions. This type of foundation gives your complexion a smooth, radiant finish.

Combination and oily skins need a water-based liquid foundation that reduces shine without drying. Choose a fragrance-free formulation that provides natural, translucent coverage.

Excessively oily skin requires an oil-free, water-based liquid foundation that's totally free of oils, waxes, and fragrance. Those with this skin type should opt for a formula with special oil-absorbing ingredients for maximum protection against oil buildup and shine. This type of foundation is also beneficial for teenagers and anyone who is acne prone.

How and When to Protect Apply foundation every morning after your moisture balance product for all-day beauty and protection. Smooth on lightly with fingertips using outward sweeping strokes, blending well especially along jawline. If using an oil-free formula, apply to one small area of the face at a time, since the water content in this type of product tends to evaporate rapidly. If more coverage is desired, reapply foundation after the first coat is dry.

Proper movement of application

Foundation gives your complexion a subtle hint of color and a smooth, even-toned finish as it protects against environmental elements. To apply, smooth over your face using upward and outward strokes. Be sure to blend especially well beyond the jawline and all the way to your hairline for a natural look that doesn't show where your foundation ends. Now you're ready to apply your glamour makeup.

$\mathcal{S}$kin Tones: Nature's Palette

A foundation — the final step in your basic skin-care program — not only protects your skin, it also provides the base for all your glamour cosmetics. The first step in selecting your foundation is determining what you want your makeup base to do. Studies show that the majority of women want a foundation that matches their natural color; the shade you choose should be as close to your skin tone as possible to blend and even out your facial colors. At other times, however, you may prefer your skin to have a bright, sun-kissed appearance. In addition, you may want to conceal minor imperfections with foundation.

The women pictured here illustrate the wide spectrum of skin tones. Their selection of foundation was

A Light/Ivory   **B** Light/Ivory   **C** Medium/Beige   **D** Medium/Beige

based on a scientific measurement of their skin color. In the top photographs the women's faces are clean; in the bottom photographs, each woman is wearing the foundation shade that comes closest to her natural tone. The color swatches show other complementary foundation shade possibilities. These alternatives can help you attain a range of looks — from covering freckles to making your complexion appear beautifully bronzed.

How do you know what shades will work for you? Because it is unlikely you will ever have your skin color measured scientifically, it is always best to try before you buy. Test foundations on your face in natural lighting. The inventory on the following pages will help you determine what you want your foundation to accomplish. With your answers as your guide, you'll be able to choose a foundation that meets your individual needs and is best suited to your skin. Your choice will lay the foundation for your most attractive beauty look.

E   Medium/Beige   F   Medium/Beige   G   Dark/Bronze   H   Dark/Bronze

Taking a Closer Look

Circle the answers that best describe your skin.

1. The overall coloring of my complexion in bright daylight is:
   A. Light/ivory.
   B. Medium/beige.
   C. Dark/bronze.

2. Overall, my complexion is:
   A. Consistent, generally even in color and texture.
   B. Darker around the eyes, nostrils, and mouth.
   C. Uneven — some blotchiness, discoloration, and/or freckling.

3. My skin type is:
   A. Dry.
   B. Normal.
   C. Combination.
   D. Oily.

4. I want my foundation to:
   A. Blend with my skin tone, for the most natural look possible.
   B. Enhance my natural skin tone and coloring, making it appear more golden or more rosy.
   C. Conceal or camouflage, veiling imperfections.

Your answer to statement 1 is your guide to finding a complementary foundation shade; however, keep in mind that more than one shade will most likely suit your skin tone. The most efficient way to select a makeup base is to try a number of colors before you make a decision.

Your answer to statement 2 indicates the amount of coverage you need from a foundation. If you answered A, you'll only need minimal concealing, most likely under the eye area. Apply concealer as directed on page 97 before putting on your foundation.

If your answer was B, you need additional help in concealing darker areas. Once again, follow the corrective techniques explained on page 97 to help even out your skin tone before applying foundation.

If you answered C, you will also want to follow the corrective procedures on page 97 to camouflage imperfections. After you've completed these steps, you'll achieve a flattering look by selecting an intermediate shade of foundation that blends the various tones in your complexion.

Your skin type, indicated in statement 3, also affects the formula of foundation that will be most beneficial. Refer to page 68 for the type best suited to your individual needs.

Statement 4 relates to what you want your foundation to achieve. If you answered A, you can attain a natural look by selecting a foundation shade that closely matches your skin tone and blends well with your complexion's subtle shadings.

Your natural coloring is an important consideration if you answered B. For a sun-warmed effect, choose a more golden shade. And for a look that's more radiant and alive, opt for a foundation with more rose in it.

If your answer is C, you'll want to master the art of corrective makeup to veil imperfections effectively. As a general rule, you can achieve the smoothest look by selecting an intermediate foundation shade.

Remember: you can accomplish the best results by experimenting with a variety of makeup shades. To ensure that you select a flattering shade, always try foundation before you buy.

Youthful, healthy-looking skin demands daily protection. Because the sun, more than any other single factor, can damage your skin, you'll want to make sure always to use a sunscreen outdoors.

Using Sunscreen

Use of a sunscreen is an important element in your daily skincare program *whenever* you are going to be exposed to sunlight. Remember that even in city settings and in the winter your skin absorbs ultraviolet radiation from the sun. If you live in a high altitude, or in an urban location where many buildings have glass or other reflective surfaces, you may have to use a sunscreen every day. Given all that is known about the damaging effects of sunlight on the skin, the best rule to keep in mind is: when in doubt, *use* a sunscreen.

Cream and lotion sunscreen formulas contain ingredients — the most common are forms of PABA — that provide a physical and/or chemical barrier to the sun's harmful ultraviolet rays. The amount of these barrier ingredients in a sunscreen determines the product's "sun protection factor," or SPF. This factor is indicated on the container of each product by an SPF number, which may range from 2 to 15. The higher its number, the greater a sunscreen's capacity to protect your skin from damaging ultraviolet radiation.

All types of skin, no matter how dark, require some degree of protection from the sun. Contrary to one popular misconception, sunscreens do not prevent tanning; rather, they reduce tanning and the unwanted effects of sunlight. Sunburn should always be avoided, and when used properly, sunscreens *do* prevent sunburn. To determine the right SPF number for the sunscreen product you should choose, refer to the chart below.

Skin's Usual Reaction to Sun*	Recommended SPF Number
Always burns easily; never tans	10 to 15
Always burns easily; tans minimally	8 to 10
Burns moderately; tans gradually to light brown	6 to 8
Burns minimally; always tans easily to moderate brown	4 to 6
Rarely burns; tans quickly to dark brown	2 to 4

* Based on the first thirty to forty-five minutes of exposure to the sun after a winter season of no such exposure.

Making It Yours

If you want to feel beautiful, investing time and effort to care for your skin pays off. You'll find you can have soft and smooth skin that radiates good health: skin that *shows* how well you care for it. All you have to do is establish your own beauty routine and devote a small amount of time to it every day.

More than any other single factor of beauty care, *consistency* will bring you glowing results. Your skin relies on what *you* do for it to help it function well and look its best. If you're erratic about taking care of it, your skin may respond erratically — possibly with breakouts or extreme oiliness or dryness. That's why it's so important to include the five steps to beautiful skin in your daily schedule — and to perform each step in the proper order:

Step 1: Cleanse The essential first step that removes makeup, surface oils, and impurities.

Step 2: Retexture The twice-a-week step that removes dry surface cells, exposing younger, newer skin. This step also improves and enhances the texture of the skin as it stimulates circulation.

Step 3: Freshen The very important step that removes any residue of previous products as it tones, softens, and conditions the skin's surface.

Step 4: Moisture Balance The vital step that helps skin maintain its optimum moisture balance by providing and holding in essential moisture, improving skin's resilience and elasticity (one of the most significant elements in keeping your skin young looking).

Step 5: Protect The final step that brings together a unique approach to skin care. Protecting your skin from environmental hazards with foundation gives it the healthful support it needs to face the day, *and* makes it look radiant and even-toned.

You can see from the chart at right how easy and convenient it is to include the five steps to beautiful skin in your daily routine. Good skin care is the essential groundwork for achieving and maintaining the best possible skin, and the basis from which to move on to exciting makeup techniques. So begin your own skin-care routine and make it work for you.

Five easy steps: cleanse, retexture, freshen, moisture balance, and protect. Put them to work for you to achieve the most radiant skin possible. Never miss a day. Never skip a step. Following the right beauty regimen, with the right beauty products, is the best way to keep your skin in optimum condition.

	Cleanse	Retexture	Freshen	Moisture Balance	Protect
When to Perform	Morning and evening.	Twice a week — after cleansing and before freshening. (Oily skin may need to retexture more often.)	Twice a day — after cleansing or masking.	Morning and evening after freshening.	Every morning to wear all day.
Function of Step	Cleanses skin thoroughly, gently, and effectively. Removes makeup, surface oils, and impurities. Smoothes and softens skin.	Exfoliates dry surface cells. Improves and enhances skin texture. Stimulates circulation. Removes impurities.	Softens, conditions, and tones the skin's surface. Further stimulates circulation. Completes the cleansing process. Balances pH of skin's surface.	Helps skin achieve its optimum moisture balance. Improves hydration and smoothness. Enhances skin's resilience and elasticity. Helps protect against damage caused by weather, wind, and climatic conditions.	Protects skin from environmental elements. Adds a subtle hint of color for a smooth, even-toned finish. Covers minor imperfections.

THREE

Glamour

Your personal style of beauty evolves naturally from effective, ongoing skin care, the basis for the excitement and glamour of makeup. The blush of glowing cheeks, the jewellike hues that add sparkle to your eyes and define and emphasize your every glance. The soft pinks, reds, or corals that add enchantment to your smile. Your makeup can be creative and expressive, a statement of your femininity, or a sultry, sizzling suggestion of your adventuresome self.

The Magic of Makeup

There's a certain mystique — an unmistakable magic — about makeup. It gives you an instant lift, a confident glow, and a vibrant energy. Cosmetics help you feel polished and put together; they let you define, highlight, and enhance your best features. Even more important, makeup lets you create a full-fashion look that's personalized and up to date, a look that reflects your style, your mood, and your way of life.

Today there are makeup colors, formulas, and application techniques to suit every need and occasion. Never before have so many appealing options been available. Almost magically, a woman looks — and feels — more attractive, more positive, more self-assured.

Makeup also has a positive effect on your psychological well-being. Psychologists have found that makeup can actually enhance a woman's self-esteem and sense of her self-worth. In two different research projects at large universities, psychologists uncovered some startling conclusions about women and cosmetics:

- Women who use makeup have greater self-confidence than those who don't.
- Women who use makeup tend to experience less social anxiety than those who don't.
- Women who do not use makeup tend to avoid social interaction.
- Women who want to affect others positively use makeup and tend to experiment with their cosmetics more often than those who don't.
- Women who use makeup regularly are more satisfied with the appearance of their faces than those who don't.
- Women who wear makeup are more outgoing and more sociable than those who don't.
- Women who wear makeup regularly can anticipate earning as much as 12 percent more than those who don't!

Makeup not only influences the way the world sees you, it has a strong and positive effect on the way you see yourself. Think about your own experience. It's difficult to deny that wearing makeup makes most of us feel better about the way we look and the ways others perceive us. Makeup gives you a finished, well-groomed look that can be as important to your business image as it is to your social life. When you take the time to apply makeup carefully and properly, you tell the world that you like the way you look and that

Let your makeup match the occasion, whether it's polished and professional for day or elegant and romantic for evening. Use cosmetics to create a mood — or to change one.

you want to be noticed; it reflects your interest in yourself and your appearance. Confidence generated by your own polished look is a big plus in many situations — it helps you create a good first impression when you apply for a job, meet new people at a party, make a sales presentation that really counts, meet your child's teacher, or go after an important contract or promotion.

Our widely varied daily activities call for a variety of makeup looks. Think of your cosmetics as clothing: a wardrobe of makeup looks to match your different beauty needs. In the following section we provide both the instruction and the inspiration to help you achieve your unique glamour look. We begin with basic daytime glamour makeup. This simple, convenient approach to makeup application and color is flexible enough to suit your daily needs and give you that polished look you want to face your world every day. Special tips for women on the go tell you how to make the transition from a soft, natural daytime look to a dramatic, sophisticated evening look.

Remember: you don't have to be born a perfect beauty to look pretty every day. The key is to experiment, be creative, and have fun with makeup and color. You'll discover that the change in your looks can change your life.

Glamour Basics

Makeup can make the difference, and in the following pages we tell you how to find your special look and keep it — beautifully. Here is a complete and simple procedure for applying makeup to guide you in creating your own personal look for basic daytime glamour. The tips and techniques are organized in the order we feel makeup is best applied, beginning with cheek and face color for an overall tone. Blusher contours your face with pretty definition, giving it a healthy glow. It also calls attention upward toward your eyes — your most expressive feature. Eye makeup adds a dramatic note and balances the effect of your cheek color. With eyebrow pencil, eye shadow, eyeliner, eye-defining pencil, and mascara you can create a total look that draws others' eyes to yours. You can shape, define, and enhance your eyes for an effect that suits your personal beauty style. Lip color and gloss complete the basic daytime look, adding luster and shine to your mouth. For each of these features we offer basic makeup guidelines plus special tips on how to make the most of various face, eye, and lip shapes. There's even a special section on color to help you learn what shades of blusher, eye makeup, and lip color are best for your coloring.

Once you've learned the glamour basics — the simple steps to your beautiful daytime look — we invite you to experiment and have some fun with an exciting plunge into the world of makeup. Beginning on page 114 we guide you through dozens of exciting and creative makeup looks. All you need are the Glamour Basics and your cosmetics — your ticket to a Glamour Adventure!

Begin your daytime Glamour Basics by adding color to your cheeks, using cream rouge and/or powder blusher. Eye shadow, in glorious shades or subdued neutral hues, contours your eyes and adds a touch of sophistication and everyday elegance.

Mascara is the final touch for spar-
kling eyes; brush it on your top
and bottom eyelashes to add color,
thickness, and length. Pull your total daytime glamour look together
with lip color, first defining the
shape of your mouth with a lip-
liner pencil, then filling in with
color and adding a final glimmer
of gloss.

Caring for Your Makeup

Almost all cosmetics that contain
coloring agents are sensitive to
ultraviolet and visible radiation;
keep them out of direct sun and
away from windows. In addition,
dampness can affect both powder-
based and cream-based makeup.
High humidity causes powders to
crumble or it may create the
ideal conditions for mold to form
on cream-based cosmetics. Cosmetics will last longer and stay
fresher if you keep them on a
vanity table in your bedroom,
rather than in the bathroom
where you shower.

Never leave cosmetics in your
car in very cold or very hot
weather. When you travel by
plane, carry your cosmetics with
you rather than packing them in
your checked luggage. Keep your
cosmetics away from drafty windows, heating ducts, or air-conditioning outlets.

Containers should always be
closed securely to protect con-
tents from dust or environmental
soils, and be sure to wash your
hands before using cosmetics.
Clean cosmetic brushes after you
use them. Lip, blending, eye,
blusher, and powder brushes
should be carefully wiped clean
with a tissue. Eye-shadow brushes
should be rinsed with tepid water
and gently dried with a tissue
when they become soiled. Once a
month wash your brushes in mild
detergent and rinse them with
tepid water. Be sure to dry them
thoroughly before storing. A cool,
dry storage place for brushes will
help them last longest.

All disposable items for makeup
application — cotton balls or cotton swabs, for example — should
be kept in closed containers to
keep them clean. Do not use
them more than once.

Taking a Closer Look

Choosing makeup colors is an important — and exciting — part of putting your glamour look together. With a bit of practice and ingenuity you can achieve any number of effects — from soft and subtle to daring and dramatic. The key is in developing your color potential: learning how to use glamour shades for maximum impact and experimenting with different color combinations and application techniques to discover those just right for you.

Before you begin, take a few minutes to think about the many ways in which color affects your life each day. Color is a way to communicate feelings, to express emotions, and to convey a mood. It's the joy of seeing . . . it's light, life, and energy. Color can be subtle, delicate as a whisper. Or it can be exuberant, exciting, and exhilarating.

Now, think about how you feel when you wear certain colors. We all have a few items in our wardrobe that make us look, and feel, sensational. Maybe it's a spectacular shade of blue that brings out the color of your eyes . . . or a pretty pastel pink that gives your complexion a soft, attractive glow. The point is, color is uniquely personal; there are no universal right or wrong choices. The trick is to understand how to use color to your best advantage — to select a shade intelligently in order to make a very real, and very appealing, difference in the way others see you . . . and the way you see yourself.

The challenge — choosing from the wide range of colors and color combinations available. In the case of glamour makeup, it's learning to use color to enhance your total look; to think of makeup color as a key fashion accessory. The ideas and tips on the following pages are designed to help you increase your color know-how and fine-tune your awareness; to provide all the information you need to change your makeup as easily — and as effectively — as you do your clothing.

Once you begin, you'll find more options and opportunities for using color than you ever imagined possible. And most important of all, you'll discover a whole new color confidence — to make changes, to experiment, and to adapt your makeup to make your own individual fashion statement.

Think of color as a key fashion accessory — to add excitement and impact to your total glamour look.

$\mathcal{Y}$our Color Vocabulary

Mastering the basics of glamour shade selection begins with an understanding of some key terms.

Hue

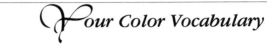

The designation of the color itself, such as red, blue, yellow, and so on.

Warm Colors

Colors with yellow, or golden, undertones.

Cool Colors

Colors with blue undertones.

Neutral

Colors that have neither yellow nor blue undertones. In addition, shades that contain just a small amount of color, and/or those that harmonize with either warm or cool colors, are often referred to as neutrals.

The definitions below will be used throughout this section on color.

Intensity

The degree of saturation or concentration in a color — or its brightness or dullness. More intense hues are vivid (a heavy concentration of color), while less intense hues are soft (a light concentration of color).

Value

The amount of lightness or darkness in a color, achieved by adding white or black.

Color Harmony

A look that is achieved by using cheek colors and lip colors from the same color family — both warm or both cool. This establishes the overall color scheme for your makeup; eye colors are then used to enhance the effect.

Taking a Closer Look

Color your world — and discover that the options for creating exciting glamour looks are unlimited. That's because there are so many shades to choose from. Blue isn't just blue ,.. it's also sky, royal, midnight, and more. Red can be ruby, brick, or rose; green might be kelly, emerald, or mint. Best of all, you can wear all of them — the key is selecting the values and intensities just right for you.

To achieve a coordinated, beautifully balanced glamour look, you need to establish the overall color scheme for your makeup — warm or cool. Most often, this is based on the color of your clothing. With a warm yellow outfit, for example, you'll want to select warm cheek and lip colors; with a cool pink outfit, cool cheek and lip colors. Simply by keeping your cheek and lip colors in the same color family as your clothing, you can create a harmonious, flattering effect.

Also important when choosing cheek and lip colors are the value and intensity of the shades you will be wearing. If you have a light skin tone, you can achieve a soft, natural look by selecting paler blushers and lip shades; if you have a darker skin tone, you'll get the same results with more intense glamour colors. When you want to create a more dramatic effect, you'll want cheek and lip shades of a contrasting intensity, either lighter or darker than your skin tone.

A third consideration in selecting a shade is to choose colors you like — those that are your personal favorites. Everyone is intuitively attracted to certain shades — and quite often, they're the shades they look best in. Have you ever noticed that you get the most compliments on days you're wearing your favorite colors? That's because your color intuition is working for you. All you need to do to complete the look is follow the guidelines for achieving color harmony — keeping cheek and lip color in the same color family as your clothing, warm or cool.

There are cases, however, when determining color family may be more difficult, particularly with pastels that contain just a small amount of color. Here, you'll want to train your eye to see warm and cool undertones; to not just look at the color itself, but to decide whether it harmonizes with other warm or cool colors. Your objective is to select makeup shades that will best enhance the out-

For a coordinated look, your blusher and lip color should harmonize with your outfit. With cool shades, choose cool cheek and lip shades.

fit in question; to choose a warm or cool color scheme based on what will look most appealing.

Other special situations — including using shades in the red family and choosing makeup colors when wearing neutrals such as black, white, and gray — are covered in the section on coordinating fashion and makeup on pages 88–89.

Once your blusher and lip color determine the overall color scheme for your makeup — warm or cool — you can then use eye shadow shades to accent and enhance your look. Here, the possibilities for creating fabulous eyes truly are endless; what's most important is your own creativity and sense of style.

Most often, your outfit will provide a starting point for choosing eye shadow shades. If possible, pick out one of the tones in your garment; then use that color as your primary shade. Next, if more color is desired, add accent shades for extra interest and impact. In situations where you don't have an eye shadow that matches your clothing, your best bet is selecting a more neutral shadow — perhaps a gray or a taupe that will give you a subtle yet flattering effect.

Eye color is another factor in selecting eye shadow shades. Here, don't match your shadow to your eyes — instead, choose colors that complement and enhance their natural beauty. The chart on page 87 provides some of the most appealing combinations; try those listed and then experiment to find the ones that work best for you.

While eye shadows do offer the most flexibility, it is important to keep the intensity of eyes, lips, and cheeks consistent. A more vibrant blush, for example, calls for equally dramatic lip and eye colors. Along these same lines, a pale lip color will look best with softer cheeks and eyes. Always keep in mind the total look you want to achieve — how all your makeup shades work together for a beautifully balanced effect.

In addition to eye shadow, eye-defining pencils and eyeliner can be used to add color, interest, and emphasis to eyes. You choose how much color to use and whether to mix or match shades for just the look you want. The Glamour Adventure looks on pages 126–135 will give you some ideas; then use your creativity to come up with more of your own.

With warm shades of clothing, select warm cheek and lip shades for a harmonious effect.

Putting It All Together

The following tips are designed to help you use color for maximum impact; to put together a coordinated glamour look easily and effectively. The key — stepping out of your comfort zone . . . being open to trying a new shade or a different technique.

As you begin experimenting with the various ideas outlined, keep in mind that these are just some of the many possibilities for wearing and combining shades. The real fun of glamour makeup is taking advantage of all the options available — and once you get started, you'll be on your way to fulfilling your color potential.

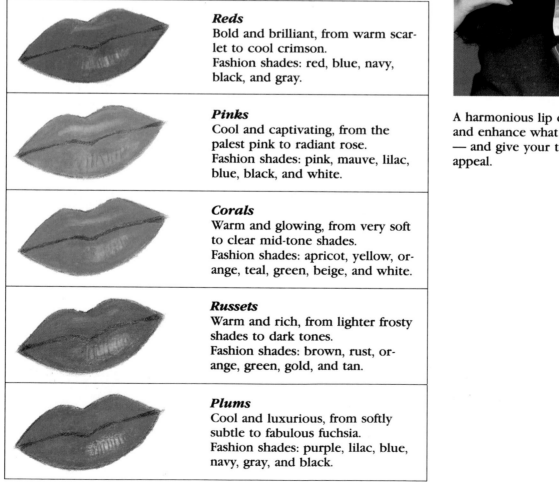

A harmonious lip color will accent and enhance what you are wearing — and give your total look instant appeal.

Reds
Bold and brilliant, from warm scarlet to cool crimson.
Fashion shades: red, blue, navy, black, and gray.

Pinks
Cool and captivating, from the palest pink to radiant rose.
Fashion shades: pink, mauve, lilac, blue, black, and white.

Corals
Warm and glowing, from very soft to clear mid-tone shades.
Fashion shades: apricot, yellow, orange, teal, green, beige, and white.

Russets
Warm and rich, from lighter frosty shades to dark tones.
Fashion shades: brown, rust, orange, green, gold, and tan.

Plums
Cool and luxurious, from softly subtle to fabulous fuchsia.
Fashion shades: purple, lilac, blue, navy, gray, and black.

The two charts below will help you use eye shadow colors for exciting results. The first chart shows you a sampling of flattering eye shadow shade combinations. Experiment with those suggested, then try some of your own to find the ones best suited to you. The second chart provides eye shadow shade recommendations that will accent and enhance the color of your eyes. Once again, this is just a starting point for creating a myriad of spectacular eye looks.

Blue Eyes	Green Eyes	Brown Eyes	Hazel Eyes
Plum	Plum	Plum	Plum
Pink	Pink	Pink	Pink
Rose	Rose	Rose	Rose
Peach	Peach	Pale Blue	Peach
Green	Teal	Deep Blue	Deep Blue
Brown	Pale Blue	Teal	Brown
Gray	Deep Blue	Green	Teal
Deep Blue		Peach	Gray
		Gray	

Brights

What makeup shades will best enhance the beautiful brights in your wardrobe? The key word here is *balance*; selecting glamour colors that will stand up to bright-colored clothes. Choose eye shadow shades of a matching intensity — exquisite jewel tones and deep rich neutrals. You'll also want to apply a more intense shade of lip color — a medium to dark shade that harmonizes with what you are wearing. This is your opportunity to go a bit brighter . . . a bit bolder with your makeup for exciting effects.

Pastels

Your prettiest pastels call for makeup applied with a lighter touch — soft, elegant shades that will give you a beautifully balanced look. Pale colors are the easiest to wear, and complementary makeup shades of the same intensity can maximize their appeal. Most important — choosing eye shadows and lip colors that accent and enhance; shades that blend or harmonize with the softness of your outfit. You'll find a lip intensity controller especially useful — simply brush on over or under your lip shade to achieve exactly the effect you desire.

Black

Every woman has her favorite little black dress — and nothing can make it more appealing than well-chosen makeup shades. Black lets you go a bit bolder, a bit more daring with your glamour look. You can wear dramatic, more intense shades for dazzling results. Still another option — working with a black value controller eye shadow. Apply under or over your choice of eye shadow shade to deepen the color. And to ensure a harmonious effect, be sure to keep blusher and lip color in the same color family — warm or cool.

Prints

Prints, plaids, stripes, and multi-colored clothing present a special challenge — but with a bit of creativity and practice you can achieve exciting effects. Let the predominant color family of your outfit — warm or cool — or the shade worn closest to your face determine the overall color scheme for your makeup. Or if warm and cool tones are equally mixed, select the color family you think will be most flattering. In addition, you may want to pick an eye shadow or lip color that matches one of the colors in your clothing; then complete your look with complementary shades that will add to the appeal.

Special Considerations: Color Harmony

Certain fashion colors require that you take extra care in choosing coordinating makeup shades. Those that do fall in the red-to-yellow spectrum of the color wheel — more specifically, red, pink, rose, orange, coral, and yellow.

Your first decision — determining color family. Here, you need to look at the undertone of the garment. With blue undertones, you'll want cool makeup colors; with yellow undertones, warm makeup colors. As a general rule, pinks and roses are cool, while oranges, corals, and yellows are warm. Reds can be tricky — a blue-red, for example, harmonizes with cool glamour shades; an orange-red, with warm glamour shades.

What makes this determination important is that using blusher and lip color from the opposing color family can detract from your total look. Pink cheek and lip shades with a coral outfit clash; you lose the attractive, harmonious effect coordinating makeup shades provide. Instead, choose a blusher and lip color that match or tone with the garment; shades in the same color family that will give you a polished, pulled-together effect.

As the examples below illustrate, properly chosen glamour shades can help you create a look that's in complete color harmony — makeup and clothing work together for truly radiant results.

A

B

C

D

Cheek colors

Eye colors

Lip colors

E

F

G

H

lusher

Blusher, the first step in your basic glamour look, gives cheeks a fresh glow of color. The shade you choose sets the overall tone for your makeup — radiantly warm or vibrantly cool.

First, you'll want to select what type of blusher to use, basing your decision on your skin type and the effect you want to achieve. The two most popular product forms are cream blush, which is especially recommended for dry to normal skin, and powder blusher, which is particularly suited for combination to oily skin, although it can be used by all skin types.

To achieve a harmonious, color-coordinated look, it's important to choose a blusher shade in the same color family as your lip color. Use the color of your clothing as a guide — with cool outfits, opt for cool cheeks and lips; with warm clothes, select warm cheeks and lips. You also want to choose a lip color that will complement your blusher — as a general rule, wear pinks and roses together; peaches, corals, and coppers together. (Refer to the section on color, pages 82–89.) For the most flattering effect, it's always best to experiment with different shades to find those that accent your look and enhance your skin tone.

To achieve a natural blush and give your face soft, natural-looking color, choose a blusher that's the same intensity as your natural skin tone. Or, if you prefer, you can brighten your complexion with a slightly more intense or vibrant shade of blusher. As you make this decision, and try out different shades, consider what you want your makeup to accomplish, the outfit you're wearing, the time of day, and the type of light you will be seen in.

For extra, long-lasting color, you can use cream blush as a base for your powder blusher. Again, you'll need to select shades in the same color family for the most flattering effect. Layered in this way, your cheek color will stay fresher longer, with minimum touch-ups necessary.

To find the hollow of your cheek, place your finger on your cheekbone where it intersects with your jawbone. Now open your mouth; you should be able to feel where the two bones are hinged. Slip your fingertip down into the area just below that intersection — that's the hollow of your cheek.

Applying Cream Blush

To apply cream blush, begin by looking straight into a well-lit mirror. Find the top ridge of your cheekbone and place a dot just below your temple. Next, moving inward along your cheekbone, place a second dot of blush at the outer edge of your eye and a third dot at the outer edge of your iris.

Your three dots should form a diagonal line on your cheekbone, as shown. Then, using a light upward motion, gently blend outward toward your hairline.

Blusher & Face Powder

Powder blusher gives your face soft, natural color with a matte finish. In addition, it can also contour, shape, slim, enhance, and draw the observer's eye upward — polishing and perfecting your overall glamour look. This product form works well with all skin types, and is particularly recommended for those with combination to oily skin.

Guidelines for applying powder blusher are covered at right. Depending on your face shape, you may want to modify some of these instructions to meet your individual needs (see pages 98–99). No matter what technique you use, however, proper blending is essential in applying blusher. The color should always fade forward — the most intense color at the top of your cheekbone, gradually softening toward the center of your face. What you want to avoid is a "racing stripe" effect, which can result from insufficient blending or improper placement of color. Also take care not to apply color too far down on the face (which can draw the observer's eye downward) or closer to the nose than the width of two fingers.

A blending or blusher brush may be helpful in creating the soft, natural look you want. Stroke the brush lightly over your blusher until your cheek color blends perfectly with your foundation.

Translucent Face Powder Applied after cream blush or rouge, and before or after powder blush, translucent face powder gives your skin a smooth, matte finish as it helps blend cheek color with your natural skin tone. You may choose from two types of powder according to your individual preference. Loose powder is most often used at home after applying your makeup, while pressed powder is ideal for touch-up throughout the day. Translucent face powder does not noticeably add to or alter the color of your foundation; it works to even out and enhance the texture of your skin. The shade of powder you choose should complement both your natural coloring and foundation shade.

For best results, apply powder over your entire face with a brush. Always use long, light strokes, working from your forehead down to your chin. For all skin types, powder gives your face a finished appearance and helps "set" foundation and cheek color. For oily skin, it also works to offset facial shine, absorb surface oil, and keep makeup looking fresh.

To apply powder blusher, gently fluff brush on blusher cake to push color up into the brush. Shake off any excess. Then, beginning where you want the most intense color — on the top of the cheekbone just under the temple — gently blend inward along the cheekbone so color fades forward.

To apply translucent powder, brush over your entire face using gentle downward strokes.

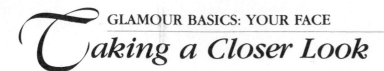

Taking a Closer Look

If you have an **average** face shape, or oval, all features are in proportion. The widest part of your face is your forehead, tapering gently from forehead to chin. This is the most common face shape, and is ideal for all makeup application techniques.

If you have a **full** face, your forehead, cheeks, and/or jawline appear wider. When applying makeup, you have a greater area to work with. Special application techniques will help you create a slimmer appearance — most important is drawing the observer's eye upward with eye makeup and properly placed blusher.

If you have a **small** face, you have small features and less facial area to work with when applying makeup. Special application techniques will help you enhance your features — most important is creating a balanced look with properly applied blusher.

Concealing and Highlighting

Before applying your foundation, you'll want to use concealer to camouflage under-eye circles, blemishes, discoloration, and minor imperfections. Concealer helps to even out your skin tone, creating a smooth, flawless finish.

For best results use a yellow concealer that's especially formulated for your individual skin type. If you have dry or normal skin, a cream concealer is recommended; for combination or oily, choose a liquid formulation. In addition, if you have a bronze, or dark, skin tone, you may want to add a touch of your foundation to your concealer for optimum coverage.

To apply, use your ring finger to lightly pat a small amount of concealer directly on those areas you want to conceal. Then, with patting movements, work outward so the concealer color becomes progressively paler.

Be careful not to overblend concealer or you will reduce its effectiveness. You also want to avoid applying too much, covering only as much of the facial area as necessary — generally not more than 20 percent of your face.

Bringing out a special area of your face is called highlighting, based on the principle that light brings out features while dark causes them to recede. You can achieve beautiful results by using a white liquid facial highlighter on top of your foundation.

Areas of your face you'll want to highlight are the browbone, along the outer half of your eyebrow; on the top of your cheekbone, below the outer corner of your eye; and on the center of your chin. As a special highlight for darker skin, also apply highlighter directly under the iris on top of the cheekbone to lighten the center of your face and enhance your eye makeup.

Application of highlighter is similar to that of concealer. Dot a small amount on the tip of your ring finger, then pat on those areas you wish to highlight. Continue patting on skin until color is blended, working up and out. Blending is particularly important in achieving the desired effect — the trick is to blend just enough to draw attention to your features without losing the effect you want. Too much highlighter can detract from, rather than enhance, your face.

Skillfully applied concealer and highlighter, in tandem with your foundation, will give you the perfect base for all your glamour cosmetics.

Taking a Closer Look

Those with an ***average*** face shape have the most flexibility in their blusher application. For a basic, natural look, begin on top of the cheekbone just under the temple, blending color inward along the cheekbone so color fades forward. You can also experiment with other application techniques outlined on pages 92–95. Experiment with various warm or cool shades to find the look most flattering for you.

If your face is ***full,*** you can create a slimming effect by starting your blusher application from a wider base, stroking from the top of the cheekbone toward the bottom of the ear. Blend inward, making sure not to bring the color too far down on your face. You can also experiment with warm or cool color schemes to find the most flattering look.

If your face is ***small,*** you want to keep your blusher in proportion for optimum balance. Stroke blusher from your temple over your cheekbone, then downward to balance your smaller facial area. Be especially careful not to bring the color in too close to your nose — never more than the width of two fingers. Try out a variety of warm or cool shades to achieve the look that's best for you.

Choosing Glasses

Eyeglasses are an important fashion accessory today. When you select eyeglass frames, be sure they are proportionate in size to your face; the upper perimeters should not extend above your eyebrows. The right frames can actually enhance the contours of your face. The secret lies in knowing how various sizes and shapes of eyeglass frames affect the way you look. Oval or circular frames help round the curves of an angular face, softening a square jaw or protruding cheekbones. Square frames add needed angles to a round or full face, giving definition to ample contours. Aviator frames — asymmetrical ovals with the broadest part resting toward the outer areas of the face below the corners of the eyes — add fullness to the lower face and give symmetry to a nar-row or pointed chin. Upswept oval frames that are widest at the temples, above the outer corners of the eyes, can make the eyes appear farther apart and the brow area broader. Such frames are flattering to a narrow face or one with a proportionally wide jaw. Wide-bridged frames create the impression of a slimmer face, especially if the outer edges of the frames extend beyond the temples. Low-bridged frames tend to shorten or minimize a long or large nose.

If you wear glasses, you'll want to take advantage of the extra attention they focus on your eyes by using the very best eye makeup techniques. Draw attention toward the lower areas of your eyes, to balance the upper eyes and brows accentuated by most cycglass frames.

If you wear eyeglasses, you'll want to use a special technique when applying blusher. Color should be applied on top of your cheekbone so it is visible both through the lenses and below the bottom of your frames. You want to avoid placing blusher below your glasses, as this will draw the observer's eye downward.

With neutral or pale glasses, the choice of blusher shade is up to you. If, however, your frames are a bright or intense color, you'll want to select a blusher shade that will enhance, not clash with, your eyeglasses.

Eyebrow Pencil

Eyebrows frame your eyes and add expression to your entire face. On most women one eyebrow has a "better" shape than the other — a more natural arc or a smoother line. Decide which of your eyebrows is better and use it as a guide for shaping the other one. The natural shape you want can be achieved by tweezing, waxing (see below), or using an eyebrow pencil.

An eyebrow pencil is used to add shape and fullness to eyebrows. It should have a fine point for easy application and soft lead for a soft, natural line. Eyebrow pencils come in a wide variety of shades, so you can select one to match your natural eyebrow coloring or hair coloring perfectly. The color should never be darker than that of your brows or hair color, unless you have very light-colored hair.

Shaping Your Eyebrows

Tweezing is an excellent way to thin brows that are too bushy. *Never* pull out hairs above the natural line of your eyebrows; tweeze only brow hairs under your eyebrows, on the bridge of your nose, or beyond the outer corners of your eyes. (Take care not to thin your eyebrows too much; the delicate hair follicles in this area can be destroyed by tweezing, and hair may not grow back.)

When you tweeze, follow the guidelines for determining eyebrow shape, as illustrated at far right. Wash your tweezers with mild detergent and rinse them well. Then dampen a facecloth with very warm water and hold it gently against the area to be tweezed; this cleans the area and opens the follicles slightly so that tweezing is easier and less painful. Look into a well-lighted mirror and tweeze out the unwanted brow hairs one at a time, rinsing the tweezers periodically to remove clinging hairs.

Another option for shaping brows is *waxing* the stray hairs that grow below the eyebrow. Don't try to do it yourself because it can be dangerous to use hot wax so near your eyes; many beauty salons offer the service at reasonable prices.

Eyebrow waxing is done by applying small amounts of liquid molten wax with a narrow brush to the area right under the brows. When the wax dries and hardens, it is peeled off, removing stray hairs by pulling them out of their follicles. The area will be red for a few hours after waxing, so it is best to wait until the following day to apply eye shadow. Because full regrowth after waxing takes about six to eight weeks, you may want to tweeze some stray brow hairs between treatments.

To apply eyebrow pencil, begin by brushing your eyebrows with an eyebrow brush, using quick, upward strokes to remove excess foundation or face powder. Brushing the hairs up also allows you to see their natural color and shape clearly. Then, with outward brush strokes, smooth the hairs in the direction in which they grow.

Now, hold your eyebrow pencil upright so it intersects the inner corner of your eye in a straight line (see photo at right and 1 in diagram below); this is where your eyebrow should begin. If yours falls short of this line, use light, short, feathering strokes of the pencil to fill in your brow.

Next, hold the pencil at an angle so it touches the outer edge of your nostril and intersects with the outer corner of your eye(2); this is where your eyebrow should end. Then hold the pencil parallel to your eye across the bridge of your nose so the inner and outer ends of your brow intersect(3). Your eyebrow should end at the same level at which it begins, or it may be slightly higher than the beginning of your brow. Your eyebrow's outer end should never droop below the inner one.

Now, hold your pencil upright, intersecting the outer edge of the iris of your eye and the middle of your eyebrow(4). This is the point at which the brow should arch highest. The end of your eyebrow, above the outer corner of your eye, should never be higher than this arch, and the ends of both brows should be on an even level.

To shape your brows properly, begin by using short, light strokes of the pencil to outline the top of each eyebrow up to its arch. Use featherlike strokes to extend each brow to the end. Fill in any sparse areas by using these same strokes, as though drawing on individual brow hairs. Then brush your brows with an eyebrow brush to smooth them and blend in the pencil strokes.

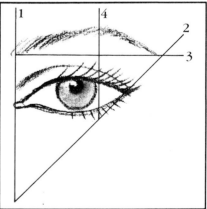

Eye Shadow

In selecting eye shadow shades, you have maximum flexibility. First, you'll want to consider what you are wearing. Eye shadows that pick up or accent one of the shades in your outfit will give a fashionable and flattering effect. Next, you should select shadows that complement your blusher and lip color for a beautifully balanced look. Still another option is wearing eye shades that bring out the color of your eyes (see the eye color chart on page 87). And finally, take into account your personal preferences — the colors you like and feel good wearing.

You will, however, want to take special care when working with eye shadows in the peach and pink ranges. For a harmonious effect, wear peach shades with warm cheeks and lips; pink shades with cool cheeks and lips. For more ideas on using and combining eye shadow shades, see the Glamour Adventure eye looks beginning on page 126.

Eye shadow instantly transforms your eyes into vibrant bouquets of color. And learning to apply eye shadow artfully is easy — with a little practice you'll soon be able to achieve a complete wardrobe of eye looks.

To help you follow the directions for eye makeup application, this diagram names the various parts of the eye area.

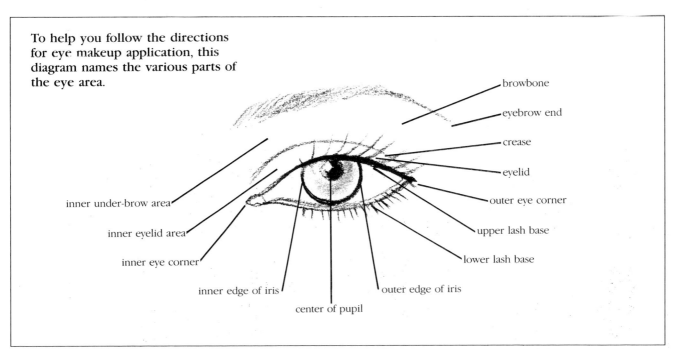

browbone

eyebrow end

crease

eyelid

outer eye corner

upper lash base

lower lash base

outer edge of iris

inner under-brow area

inner eyelid area

inner eye corner

inner edge of iris

center of pupil

ye Shadow

For your basic eye look, you need:
- a pale highlighter shade to accent and enhance
- your choice of eye shadow shade to color and contour
  In addition, you'll want to have the right tools at hand:
- a sponge-tip applicator or a soft, straight-bristled eye shadow brush to apply shadow
- a full, round-bristled brush about one half inch wide for blending eye shadow

Pressed powder eye shadow is the most commonly used product form. It can be applied dry, with a sponge-tip applicator, or wet, with a brush. To apply dry, color can be easily controlled for a beautifully blended look. Gently touch the sponge-tip applicator to the cake; then sweep shadow onto your eye, tapering and blending as you go. If applying shadow wet, dampen your brush and mix shadow to a smooth consistency; then stroke on your eye using a quick back-and-forth motion. The more water you use, the less intense your shadow color will be. Wet or dry, always use a blending brush to carefully blend one shade into the other.

A combination of the above instructions will give your eye shadow extra staying power. Simply apply eye shadow dry as instructed above; then, use a slightly dampened glamour blending brush to blend and set the color.

Finally, you may also want to try a special type of eye shadow — called a value controller — to vary the intensity of your look. These are black and white eye shadows that you apply under or over any shade of shadow to create just the effect you desire. Again, blending is important for a smooth, natural look.

For the basic glamour eye look pictured at right, use a sponge-tip applicator or eye shadow brush to apply highlighter across your lid and browbone, from lashline to brow. Next, apply your choice of eye shadow shade — first, along the upper lashline, beginning above the iris and extending to the outer corner; then upward above the crease onto the browbone and inward along the crease to the center of the iris, forming a V–shape. Blend well to avoid any harsh lines.

ye Definers

To line, define, and accent your eyes, use eye-defining pencils and liquid eyeliners. Both are available in a range of shades to beautifully enhance your finished look. In addition, eye definers accentuate the shape of your eyes and make your lashes look thicker.

In selecting what shades of eye-defining pencils and eyeliners to use, consider what effect you want to create. Brown or gray will give you the most natural look; black will provide a more striking appearance. You can also define your eyes with rich, radiant color, mixing and matching with your eye shadow shades.

Because lining and defining your eyes requires precision and control, you'll want to practice the techniques outlined on these two pages. Once you master the basic application procedure, you'll make eye defining a regular part of your glamour makeup.

Eye-defining pencils add definition and a hint of color to your eyes. The pencil should have a fine point and a medium to soft lead so it glides on easily. (It's a good idea to have a sharpener you use only for your eye-defining pencils, to keep the points sharp and the tips clean.) To apply, lightly stroke a single fine line at the base of your upper eyelid, from inner to outer corner. Next, draw another fine line just under the lower lashes, from outer to inner corner. To soften or smudge the line, use a cotton swab or an angled eye brush.

The *eyeliner* you choose should have a quick-drying, smudge-resistant liquid formula. Also select one that comes with a finely tapered brush for easiest application.

As you extract the eyeliner brush from its tube, wipe off any excess on the lip of the tube. Then, using the tip of the brush, start at the inner corner of the upper lashline and pull color evenly and gently across to the outer corner — keeping the brush as close to the lashes as possible. You can also apply liquid eyeliner under the lower lashes, stroking color from outer to inner corner.

If you find this technique is difficult to do, you may want to try applying eyeliner with short strokes instead of one continuous line. In addition, you can also experiment using liquid eyeliner and eye-defining pencil for the same eye look — use the eyeliner above the upper lashes, the eye-defining pencil under the lower lashes. Finally, for a more dramatic look, you can use the side of your eyeliner brush — rather than the tip — to create a slightly thicker line.

Mascara

Your eyelashes softly frame your eyes, and adding mascara darkens and thickens your lashes to give your eye makeup the finishing touch. Many women consider mascara to be *the* essential makeup they wear — no matter what the occasion. And it's easy to understand why. Mascara softly accentuates the natural shape and setting of your eyes, bringing out their color and expressiveness.

Mascara packaged in a tube with a fine spiral brush applicator is easy to apply; it curls your eyelashes as it adds color and fullness. Select a neutral shade of mascara — a brown or black — that's compatible with your coloring. Some women make the common mistake of choosing a mascara that's too dark. If your lashes are brown and your eyes are pale, deep black mascara can look harsh and detract from the softness your eyes should convey. Mascara should darken your eyelashes, not change their natural color.

Even smudge-resistant and waterproof mascara may wear off a bit during the day. An occasional extra touch of mascara on the tips of your lashes can do wonders to brighten up your look, so carry your mascara with you wherever you go. For best results, always keep the cap securely closed to keep the mascara from drying out and to prevent contamination, and never share mascara with anyone.

Apply mascara by looking straight into your mirror, with your chin lifted slightly so you can see your lashes clearly. Open your mouth a bit to relax your face. Supporting your elbow on a table or vanity while you apply the mascara helps keep your hand steady.

Gently twist the spiral brush as you withdraw it from the tube case. Never pump your mascara brush up and down in the tube; this distributes the mascara unevenly on the brush and often breaks its bristles. It can also dry out the mascara faster. Stroke your upper lashes evenly from their base to the tips, curling them upward with the brush as you apply the mascara. If your lashes are very light in color you may want to begin applying mascara to the tips, then stroke the lashes from underneath. The initial application to the tips may help you see the lashes better.

Reinsert the brush in the tube and apply mascara to your lower lashes with downward strokes, wiggling the brush back and forth a bit to separate the lashes. After you have applied the mascara to both eyes, you can repeat the application to add more fullness to your eyelashes. If your eyelashes are thick and grow close together, they may clump together when you apply mascara. Allow the mascara to dry, then use the corner of your eyebrow brush to carefully separate your eyelashes.

If your eyelashes are difficult to curl, you may want to consider using an eyelash curler. Use it gently after each application of mascara.

Removing Waterproof Mascara

Waterproof mascara is practical for many active women. It has more holding power than the regular formula, which is beneficial if you live in a hot, humid climate or if you like to swim with your makeup on. Because waterproof mascara is not water soluble, it might not come off with your normal cleansing routine. To take it off in the evening before cleansing your face, it is necessary to use a special oil-based, water-proof-mascara remover to dissolve the mascara gently while conditioning your lashes and surrounding skin.

To remove waterproof mascara, apply a small amount of remover to a piece of sterile cotton or a clean cotton ball. Then, very gently, wipe the cotton over each closed eye, stroking downward and outward. Continue to apply the remover until the cotton shows no traces of mascara. Always stroke very lightly and in a downward direction; this reduces the chances of the runover getting into your eye. Then open your eye and look up, to remove any traces under your lower lashes. Never rub back and forth against your lashes, as this can pull some out and damage the fragile skin on your eyelids.

Next, proceed to your skin cleansing routine. Your cleanser will pick up any remover that remains around your eyes. Close your eyes and rinse them gently by splashing on tepid water with your fingertips. Pat your eyes lightly with a clean towel to dry them.

aking a Closer Look

There is a great amount of potential for enhancing what is unique about your eyes. This inventory is designed to help you identify the specific shape of your eyes so you can use special makeup techniques to bring out their beauty.

Every woman should be able to experiment with *every* glamour eye makeup technique, not only those dictated by the shape of her eyes. Begin by looking at the illustrations here to find the eyes that most resemble yours in shape. Then read the special tips on page 111 for adjusting the Glamour Basics eye makeup techniques to match your eyes.

Average eyes are almond in shape with an upswept lift at the outer corner. Some eyelid and crease are visible. This is the most common eye shape, and no special application techniques are necessary.

Hooded eyes are set so the natural crease is hidden and very little lid is visible. Those with this eye type may also have excessive flesh under the browbone. Special application techniques can be used to help add dimension and contour.

Deep-set eyes seem to recede because the crease of the eye is set back. Special application techniques can be used to help bring this type of eye forward.

For average eyes, apply your basic shadow as directed on page 104.

For hooded eyes, extend your choice of eye shadow shade up to your eyebrow at the outer corner; then blend inward. This extra lift will make shadow more noticeable and give hooded eyes added emphasis and dimension.

For deep-set eyes, use a slightly heavier application of your highlighter shade. Then extend your choice of eye shadow shade up over your browbone before bringing color inward. You may also want to use a darker shade of eye-defining pencil and two coats of mascara.

111

Lip Color

Lip color — the final step in your basic glamour makeup — pulls your finished look together. The shade you choose should harmonize with your blusher — both warm or both cool. Together, your blusher and lip color set the tone for your makeup; eye shadow will accent and enhance it. The end result — a beautifully polished, color-coordinated effect.

There is a wide range of lip colors to choose from. Along with selecting a shade from the same color family as your blusher, you also want to base your selection on your skin tone, clothing, and, of course, personal preference. Those with lighter skin tones will get the most natural-looking makeup by choosing a lighter lip color; those with darker skin tones will get this same effect using a darker lip shade. You may also want to choose a lip color that picks up or tones with one of the shades in your outfit — a shade that blends and balances with what you are wearing.

Lip color is also affected by certain fashion trends. One season, light, barely there shades may be in style; the next, bold, bright reds are emphasized. While this will inevitably influence your selection, keep in mind the overall effect you want to achieve.

To help you create exactly the shade of lip color you desire, try using a neutral intensity controller. This product is especially formulated to be applied over or under your lip shade to lighten the color. As a result, you can get a variety of effects with a single lip color.

To apply lip color, begin by lining and defining the shape of your lips with a lip-liner pencil. Next, brush on creamy lip color. And finally, if you want to give your lips extra shine, add a shimmer of lip gloss.

Your **lip-liner** pencil should be slim and have a soft, pointed tip to help you control application. The color of the pencil should complement and blend with your lip shade. Apply lip-liner pencil carefully, following the natural contours of your mouth to keep your lip color from blurring or bleeding beyond your lips. Starting at the center of your upper lip, apply pencil using featherlike strokes, working toward each corner. Repeat on the lower lip, first drawing a short line in the center, then extending outward to each corner to complete the line.

To apply creamy **lip color**, stroke your lip brush firmly and evenly across the color. Then, with your mouth relaxed and lips closed, gently fill in your upper and lower lip. The color should look rich, radiant, and moist — never heavy or caked.

Lip gloss packaged in a tube with a sponge-tip applicator wand is easiest to use. Depending on the look you want to achieve, choose a natural gloss for a clear shine, or a tinted gloss for a sheer frost. Also select a formula that moisturizes lips and provides a protective sunscreen. To use lip gloss, twist the applicator wand slightly in its container so the sponge tip picks up a good amount of gloss. Dot the gloss in the center of your lower lip, then let the natural movement of your lips distribute it evenly.

Taking a Closer Look

Shape and color play equally important roles in creating the loveliest lips. As the illustrations on the following page show, you can use lip-liner pencil to create subtle illusions — thin lips will appear fuller, full lips will appear thinner.

In addition, the tips outlined below will help you use lip color for maximum impact.

Lip Tips

- For longer-lasting lip color, choose a creamy, moisturizing formula. After applying lip-liner pencil and lip color, blot with a tissue; then reapply lip color. Color will stay looking fresh.
- Give lips extra emphasis by filling in the outer corners with lip-liner pencil.
- For a soft, sheer look, use lip-liner pencil and a tinted lip gloss. Blend with a clean lip brush.
- To protect lips from the sun, choose a lip gloss that contains added moisturizers and sunscreen.
- Personalize your lip color with a lip intensity controller. For just a pale tint of color, wear intensity controller alone with lip-liner pencil. Or apply before or after your lip color to soften and lighten the shade to exactly the intensity you desire.
- For extra appeal, concentrate lip color on the outside edge of your lips. Bring lip color together with lip gloss.

- Use lip color to your best advantage. Bold colors will give smaller lips extra emphasis; softer, more muted shades will help minimize larger lips.
- For the most even and accurate application of lip color, always use a lip brush. This essential makeup tool is also a terrific way to multiply your color options — simply use your brush to blend two (or more) shades into a totally new, and flattering, lip color.
- A lip compact lets you conveniently carry your lip colors for midday touch-ups. Choose one with a mirror and lip brush for optimum versatility.
- The best way to test lip color before buying — on your lips with a clean, disposable brush. This will give you the most accurate idea of how the shade will blend with your natural skin tone.

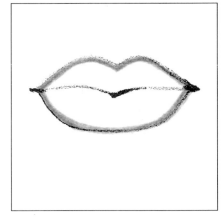

Average lips are naturally symmetrical. Apply lip-liner pencil along your natural lip line.

Thin lips will appear fuller if you apply lip-liner pencil just outside your natural lip line.

Full lips will appear thinner if you apply lip-liner pencil just inside your natural lip line. Use a slightly thicker line to further help slim lips.

Making It Yours

You're looking great — you've learned the daily basics of perfect makeup application that make your cheeks glow with soft color, give subtle definition and shimmering accents to your eyes, and shape and brighten your lips with color. This is the look you want to wear every day, knowing it makes you feel good about yourself. You're confident, groomed, polished, and professional: ready to face the day with the beautiful sense of well-being that comes from looking just right.

And it's so easy to achieve your personal makeup look when you know the best techniques for creating your prettiest face. The Glamour Basics give you a personal system for everyday glamour, a look you can always rely on, a style you can trust to work for you all day long.

Now that you know the basics, why not go even further? Why not extend and expand on what you've learned and take your looks to the limit? Why not aim for the ultimate in dazzling glamour, makeup looks you can wear when your needs go beyond the everyday?

You're now ready to pursue the next level of your beauty potential. You're ready for...

That just-right look of daytime glamour — pretty, polished, and instantly appealing. Knowing you look your best gives you the confidence to face the day — beautifully.

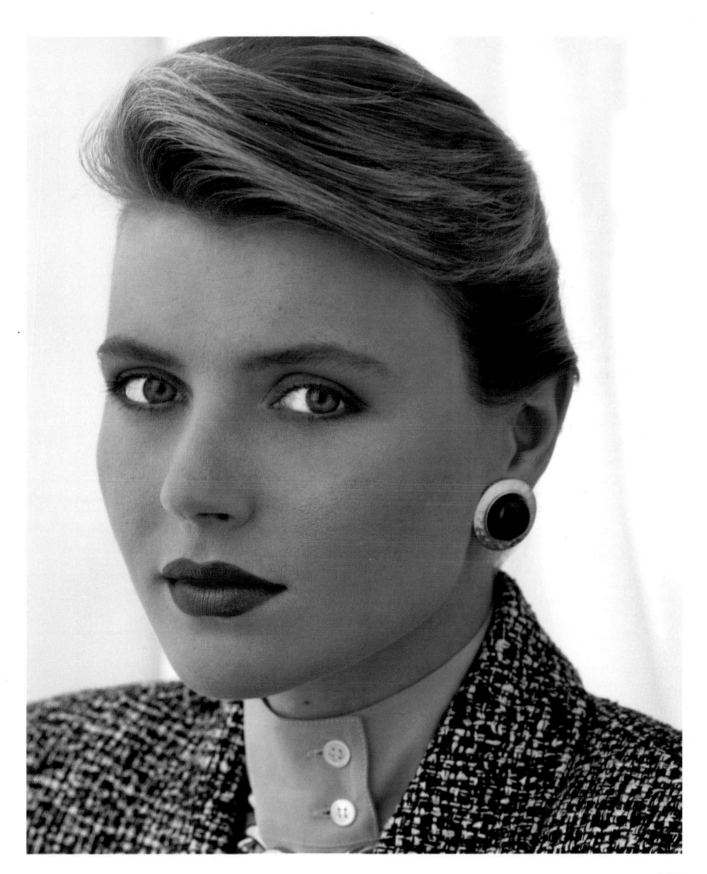

Glamour Adventure

It's an adventure into fabulously exciting makeup techniques, an exploration of your own potential to discover how beautiful you really can be simply by trying what you've never tried before. Go beyond everyday good looks and set your sights on what's different, daring, and dazzling. Take what you've learned from the Glamour Basics and add a sprinkling of sizzle, a dash of drama, a sweep of sophistication, or an exotic flourish of mystery. It's all here — a step-by-step guide to the new beauty discoveries that will take you beyond the basics into the realm of unforgettable glamour magic!

The Glamour Adventure contains an array of glamour looks that everyone can experiment with, looks designed to help you explore a wonderful variety of cosmetic techniques and colors. The Glamour Adventure will show you new looks to try with that fabulous new dress you just bought or that exciting new haircut you're planning to get. It will teach you new makeup styles for a change in the seasons, a change in your career, or a change in your mood.

Take an hour by yourself or ask a friend to join you in this adventure of new beauty experiments. Try every look — from the most dramatic to the most demure, from the most dynamic to the most spectacularly subtle. And explore your character while you're exploring the potential of your looks. You're sure to discover many delightful surprises — beautiful new ideas that work for you. Be different. Be daring. Be positively dazzling!

Change polish to pizzazz — because a glamour adventure awaits you! Be creative. Experiment. Discover how you can turn a simple daytime look into one that's simply sensational.

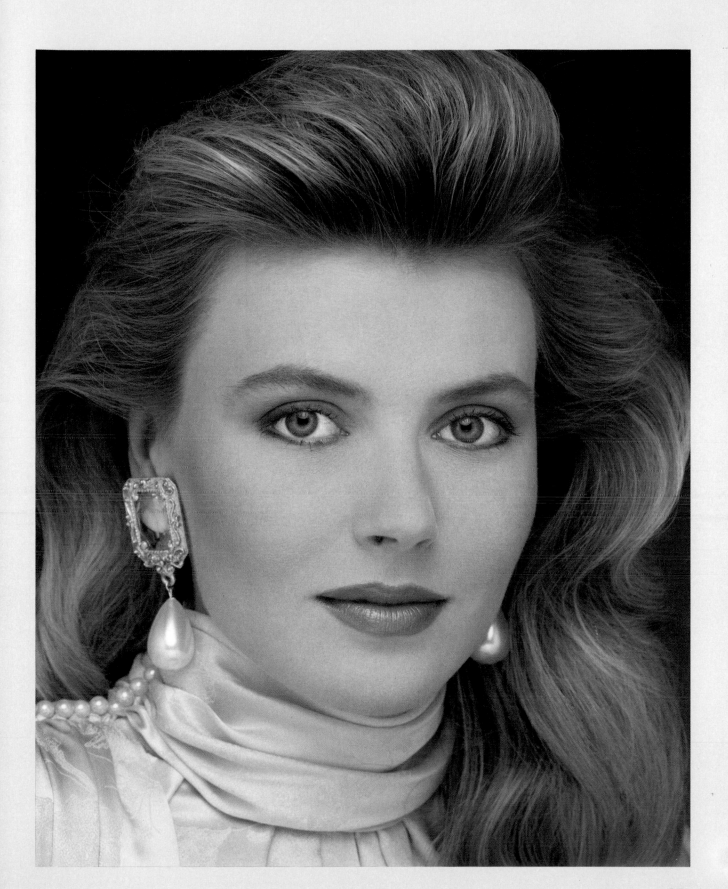

Taking a Closer Look

Makeup is magic. It can change the way you look, both to yourself and to the world. Everyday becomes exciting. Neat becomes a knockout. And simple becomes simply sensational.

The inventory below was designed to get you thinking about the reasons you wear makeup: the way it makes you feel and the effect it has on others. It is also meant to make you think about new ways you can experiment with makeup. You've already seen what basic daytime makeup can do. But why stop there? There are so many opportunities to create enchantment and illusion.

Your answers to the following questions can open your eyes to a Glamour Adventure, an experience in which you can learn how to enhance your best features and be your very own makeup artist.

1. What do you think makeup can do for you?
2. Do you enjoy putting on and experimenting with makeup?
3. Do you wish you knew how to apply makeup better?
4. Do you own a variety of cosmetics?
5. How often do you buy new cosmetics?
6. Before you put on your makeup, do you think about:
   where you are going?
   whom you are going to see?
   what you are going to wear?
   what lighting you are going to be seen in?
   what image you would like to convey?
7. Which of your features do you like best?
8. Which feature do people compliment most often?
9. What colors do you wear to make you feel terrific? (You may want to refer to pages 84 and 85.)

How you feel about makeup most likely reflects how comfortable you are using it and how receptive you are to trying new ideas. Look over your answers, then find the group or groups on these pages that best describe your "makeup personality."

If you're the type who thinks makeup is fun . . . you're probably used to changing your makeup look according to the occasion: where you are going and whom you are going to see. You know how to make your look romantic and feminine, natural and outdoorsy, or daring and bold. For you, makeup expresses a mood and conveys a desired image. Most likely, you own a wide assortment of cosmetics, but that doesn't mean you wouldn't love another new lip or eye color. That's because you enjoy wearing makeup — and it shows.

If you're the type who usually sticks with one basic makeup look . . . maybe it's time to expand your glamour outlook. If you hesitate to vary your look because of your application skills, don't despair. Set aside time to practice with the glamour ideas on the following pages. Or call on a professional beauty consultant for assistance. With some proper guidance and a bit of creativity, you soon will master a wardrobe of makeup styles. And that means you can change your look as often — and as easily — as you change your clothes!

If you're the type who's afraid of looking too "made up" . . . don't be scared off by new ideas. You can look naturally dazzling by controlling the intensity of the colors that you use. (See pages 82 to 85 for more on color and intensity.) Also keep in mind that light has an effect on the balance and tone of color, and that means your makeup can look considerably different depending on the lighting conditions. Because dimmer evening lights can drown out color, your nighttime makeup should be more dramatic and intense. The same holds true for the type of occasion: whereas festive parties call for more daring and adventurous makeup, a candle-light dinner needs a soft and very feminine touch.

If you're the type who will try any-thing once . . . terrific! The Glam-our Adventures on the following pages are tailor-made for you. Try the unexpected: colors you've never worn before, techniques that will give your look a whole new sparkle. Go for the effect — simple and sweet one day, sultry and so-phisticated the next. There's no limit to the looks — and images — you can create.

If you're the type who thinks glam-our makeup is only for the glamor-ous . . . it's time to change your thinking. Take note of your best fea-tures, the ones you like as well as those others compliment, and learn to enhance them. Take a creative approach to makeup, using ideas from the following pages. Once you become familiar with the tech-niques, you'll discover how makeup can add a new dimension to your life. And before long, you're likely to find you're among the glamor-ous, too!

If you find yourself using the same makeup colors . . . you need to ex-periment with some of the other wonderful shades available. Think about the cheek, eye, and lip colors that you use often because they complement your natural tones. Write down two cheek, eye, and lip colors you've always wanted to try:

Cheek colors _____

_____

Eye colors _____

_____

Lip colors _____

_____

In the pages to come, make a point of experimenting with these colors — and others!

Makeup Tools

To make the most of your Glam-our Adventure, be sure you have the following makeup products and tools within easy reach:

- A well-lighted mirror in which you can see yourself clearly; a lighted makeup mirror, which has several different lighting ef-fects, is ideal.
- Cleansing cream or cleanser, freshener, tissues, cotton, and a clean face-cloth dampened with warm water to remove makeup when you want to try the next technique and clean up mistakes you might make while practic-ing.
- Several shades of cream blush and powder blushers — warm and cool, light to dark — and a blusher blending brush.
- A range of eye shadows in-cluding highlighters, neutrals, and fashion colors. Include a range of different hues as well as lighter and darker shades. You'll also need sponge-tip applicators (or brushes) and an eye shadow blending brush.
- A range of eye-defining pen-cils to complement your eye shadows, eyeliner, and mascara. Also, eyebrow pencil, a brow brush, and an eyelash curler.
- An assortment of lip colors — warm and cool, light to dark — and a lip intensity controller; one or two lip-liner pencils that blend with your lip colors; and lip gloss. Also, lip brushes for color application and one lip brush for blending.

Chic Cheeks

Blusher effectively colors and contours your cheeks, giving your glamour look an overall glow. Although it's one of the simplest steps in your makeup, it's also one of the most important. Properly applied cheek color makes your face come alive; it gives you a fresh, healthy, radiant appearance. In addition, blusher pulls your look together and sets the tone for your makeup — wonderfully warm or vibrantly cool.

On these two pages, color and technique both play a part in blusher application. Most important when applying cheek color is choosing a shade that blends well with your natural skin tone. You'll also want to consider what you are wearing, making sure the shade enhances and harmonizes with the color worn closest to your face. Finally, when using more than one shade, be sure to stay within a single color family — warm or cool.

Once you master the steps needed to create each look, experiment with different shade combinations to find the ones that work best for you.

Bronzed and Beautiful

For longer-lasting cheek color, and a beautifully radiant glow, try layering your blusher — powder over cream. Begin by applying cream blush — here, a warm sandalwood — in three dots on your cheekbone: just below the temple, at the outer edge of the eye, and at the outer edge of the iris. Gently blend outward toward your hairline. Next, apply a coppery shade of powder blusher, beginning on top of the cheekbone, brushing color inward. Use a blusher brush to carefully blend the two shades.

Pretty and Polished

Two shades of powder blusher are used to accent your cheekbones and give your face a beautifully contoured look. First, apply a light pink blusher on the top of your cheekbones, beginning just under the temple where you want the most intense color to be. Brush inward using light strokes, so the color fades forward as you move closer to your nose. Next, apply a slightly darker shade in the hollow of your cheek, blending upward and outward into the lighter color. Make sure there are no lines or hard edges — you don't want to see where one shade ends and the next one begins.

Soft and Sunny

Look like you've been in the sun (even if you haven't) with this easy technique. First, apply a glowing apricot powder blush on top of the cheekbone, brushing inward so the color fades forward. Then add an extra touch of blush where the sun would hit naturally — above the brows and on the tip of the nose and chin. (To give your face a "tanned" look, you may also want to use a slightly darker shade of foundation or mix a few drops of a bronze shade to your regular color.)

Enticing Eyes

There's no denying it — a woman's eyes are her best beauty asset. Admirers focus on eyes that are alive, bright, and rich with splendid color. Eyes that are expressive and memorable. Eyes that make a lasting impression.

The simplest and most dramatic way to enhance your appearance — to add sparkle and excitement to your looks — is to play up your eyes. The skillful application of eye makeup is, in a sense, an art. It's a way to express your feelings, your mood, your sense of style. In the Glamour Adventure for eyes, you'll learn how to use color creatively; how to shape, highlight, line, and define your eyes.

Best of all, you can achieve all the looks described in the following pages — no matter what size and shape *your* eyes are. All you have to do is read the instructions, which are for almond-shaped eyes, then follow the variations recommended for your type of eye. (Refer to your eye shape inventory on pages 110 and 111.)

Try the colors suggested here. Or, if you prefer, experiment with your personal favorites. The key is to have fun, and to make beautiful eyes a natural part of you. There are no wrong or right looks for anyone, so try them all and take time to get used to the glamorous you they create.

Before you begin your Glamour Adventure, take a look at the eye shadows in your collection and decide which category each falls into. Also, your choice in both eyeliner and mascara should be compatible with your natural eyelash color, either brown or black. And as a general rule, eye-defining pencils should match the *basic* color of eye shadow used for each look, unless otherwise specified. From there it's up to you. You decide the colors, the combinations, and the intensities that will bring about the glamorous effects you desire!

The eyes have it — and here is your chance to be truly creative. Your options are unlimited — be bold and dramatic one day, romantic and feminine the next. You decide. In the Glamour Adventure you'll find eye-appealing looks to suit every mood and occasion.

Watercolor Eyes

These are soft, shimmering eyes, flirty and very feminine. The palette: pure, pale, and glowing. Pastels have never been so appealing. The key is to carefully blend shades together so there are no hard edges. Each color seems to "melt" into the next for a gentle blending of tones.

Here, Watercolor Eyes are created with pale blue, pink, shell, and orchid shadow; brown eye-defining pencil; and brown mascara.

Step 1

Step 2

Step 3

Step 4

Hooded eyes

Deep-set eyes

Step 1: Apply a wash of shell eye shadow from lashline to brow.

Step 2: Apply pale pink eye shadow to the inner third of the lid, from lashline to just above the crease. Next, apply pale blue eye shadow to the middle third of the lid, from lashline to just above the crease. Blend well. Colors should "melt" into one another; you want to overlap, but not cover, the shell eye shadow already on your lid.

Step 3: Apply pale orchid shadow to the outer third of the eye, from lashline to just above the crease; then, bring color down under the lower lashes to the outer edge of the iris. Blend well.

Step 4: Apply a thin line of brown eye-defining pencil above upper lashes and under lower lashes. Brush on one coat of brown mascara.

For hooded eyes: In step 2, extend pink and blue eye shadows up almost to the brow. In step 3, extend orchid eye shadow up to the outer corner of the brow.

For deep-set eyes: In step 1, use pink eye shadow as your wash from lashline to brow. In step 2, use shell eye shadow on the inner third of your lid (instead of pink). In step 4, apply a slightly thicker line of eye-defining pencil along upper lashline.

127

Broadway Eyes

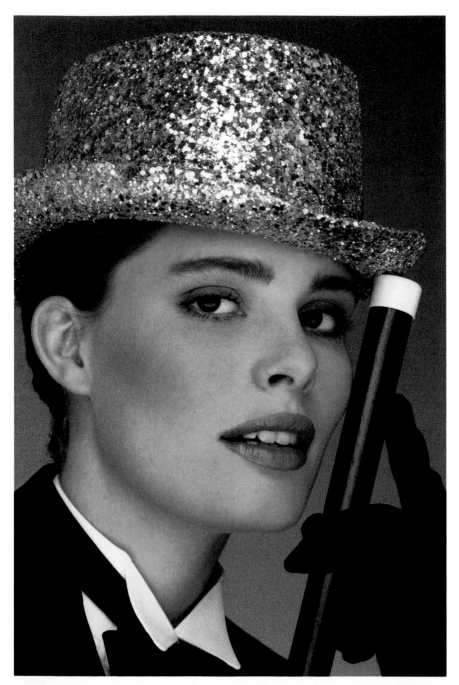

With these eyes, the spotlight is definitely on you! The world is your stage and you're the star of the show. Broadway Eyes take top billing . . . and the reviews are always terrific.

To create this show-stopping look, one vibrant eye shadow shade plays off a pair of rich naturals. Here, peach and cocoa are accented with a jolt of tantalizing teal. To further enhance the look, use brown eye-defining pencil and black mascara.

Step 1

Step 2

Step 3

Step 4

Hooded eyes

Deep-set eyes

Step 1: Apply a wash of peach eye shadow from lashline to brow.

Step 2: Apply cocoa eye shadow in the crease. Blend.

Step 3: Apply teal eye shadow in a thick line along upper lashline from the inner edge of the iris to the outer corner of the eye. Next, bring teal upward above the crease onto the browbone, then inward along the crease to just above the inner edge of the iris. Finally, bring teal down under the lower lashes from the outer corner of the eye to the outer edge of the iris.

Step 4: Apply brown eye-defining pencil above upper lashes and below lower lashes. Brush on two coats of black mascara.

For hooded eyes: In step 2, extend cocoa eye shadow up above the crease. In step 3, extend teal eye shadow to the outer edge of the brow before bringing color inward along the crease.

For deep-set eyes: In step 2, extend cocoa eye shadow up above the crease. In step 4, apply a slightly thicker line of brown eye-defining pencil above upper lashes.

rivate Eyes

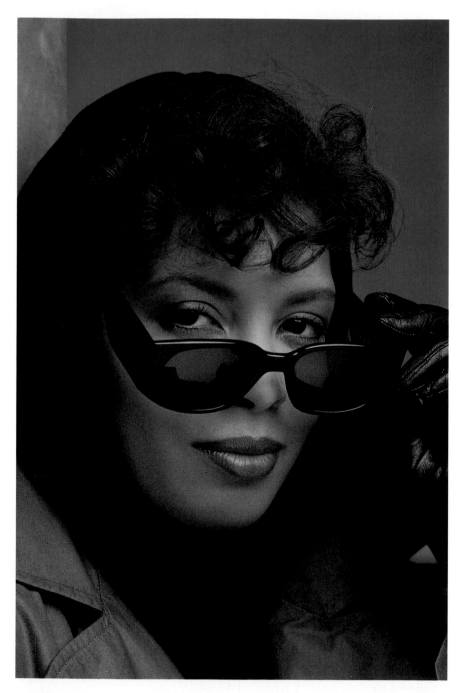

These are smoky, sultry eyes; a look for your mystical, magical moods. There's no turning back when you wear Private Eyes . . . and what you uncover is totally up to you!

To achieve this very special look, use a black eye shadow (called a value controller) over a colored eye shadow shade — here, an irresistibly appealing mauve. The trick is carefully blending to create a subtly sensual effect. Also used on these Private Eyes — shell and gray eye shadow, black eyeliner, and black mascara.

Step 1

Step 2

Step 1: Apply shell eye shadow on the browbone, just under the brow. Apply mauve eye shadow to the lid, from lashline to crease.

Step 2: Apply black eye shadow over the mauve on the outer third of the lid to form a wedge shape. Blend well to achieve just the intensity you desire. (Begin with just a small amount of black, adding more if you want a darker tone.) Also apply black under lower lashes from the outer corner to the outer edge of the iris.

Step 3: Apply gray eye shadow in the crease. Blend.

Step 4: Apply a thin line of black eyeliner along upper lashline and below lower lashes. Brush on two coats of black mascara.

Step 3

Step 4

Hooded eyes

Deep-set eyes

For hooded eyes: In step 1, extend mauve eye shadow up above crease. In step 3, apply gray eye shadow slightly above the mauve.

For deep-set eyes: In step 1, omit shell eye shadow. In step 3, apply gray eye shadow from crease to browbone. In step 4, apply a slightly thicker line of black eyeliner along upper lashline.

131

Color-Kissed Eyes

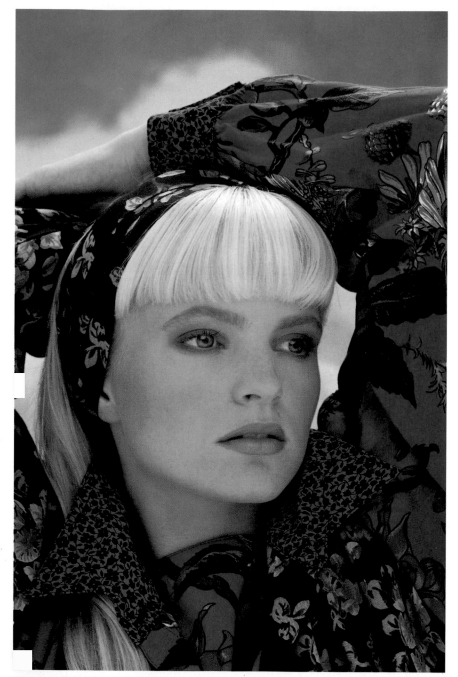

These are eyes that capture the coming of spring . . . an enticing bouquet of fresh, lively color. Color-Kissed Eyes are rich, radiant, and very romantic; a look you'll wear to enhance the mood — or to create one.

To achieve the effect, use a light and a medium tone of two different eye shadow shades — here, pinks and violets. The finishing touch — grape eye-defining pencil and black mascara.

Step 1

Step 2

Step 3

Step 4

Hooded eyes

Deep-set eyes

Step 1: Apply a wash of pale pink eye shadow from lashline to brow.

Step 2: Apply rose eye shadow in the crease and under the lower lashes from outer to inner corner. Next, apply a pale orchid eye shadow to the outer half of the lid. Blend well.

Step 3: Apply a deeper violet eye shadow just above the crease from the outer corner to the inner edge of the iris. Blend well.

Step 4: Apply grape eye-defining pencil above upper lashes and under lower lashes. Brush on two coats of black mascara.

For hooded eyes: In step 3, extend the deep violet eye shadow above the crease almost to the brow. In step 4, apply a thinner line of grape eye-defining pencil above upper lashes.

For deep-set eyes: In step 1, apply the pale pink eye shadow to the lid from lashline to crease. In step 3, extend the deep violet eye shadow up to the brow. In step 4, apply a slightly thicker line of grape eye-defining pencil along upper lashline.

Calypso Eyes

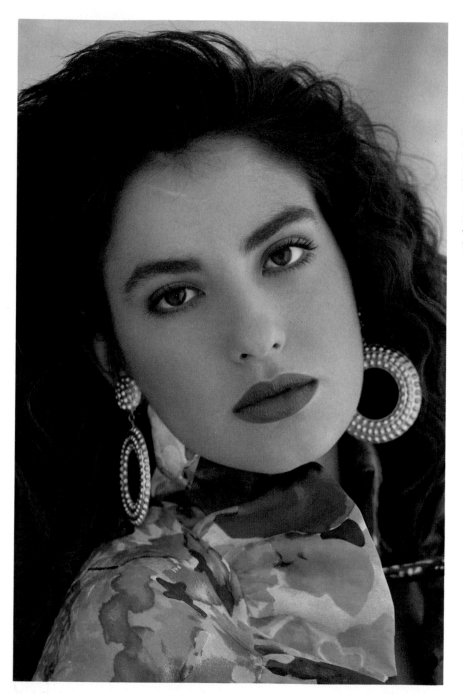

This is a look that's definitely hot; eyes that capture the glamour and excitement of your very own tropical paradise. The mood is exotic . . . the passion, intense. When you wear Calypso Eyes, the heat is on!

To achieve the effect, use a light and a deeper shade of a jewel-toned eye shadow — here, two beautiful blues. And for extra appeal, rose eye shadow on the browbone and a touch of orchid eye shadow under the lower lashes. Finally, complete the look with navy eye-defining pencil and black mascara.

Step 1

Step 2

Step 3

Step 4

Hooded eyes

Deep-set eyes

Step 1: Apply rose eye shadow on the browbone just under the brow. Next, apply pale blue eye shadow on the lid. Blend.

Step 2: Apply a deeper shade of blue eye shadow in a V-shape to both the inner and outer corners of the eye. Blend well.

Step 3: Apply orchid eye shadow under the lower lashes; smudge using a cotton swab.

Step 4: Apply a thin line of navy eye-defining pencil above upper lashes and below lower lashes. Brush on two coats of black mascara.

For hooded eyes: In step 2, apply the deeper blue eye shadow in a wider V-shape at inner and outer corners, extending color up above crease.

For deep-set eyes: In step 2, apply the deeper blue eye shadow in a wider V-shape at inner and outer corners, extending color up above crease. In step 4, apply a slightly thicker line of navy eye-defining pencil above upper lashes.

135

Luscious Lips

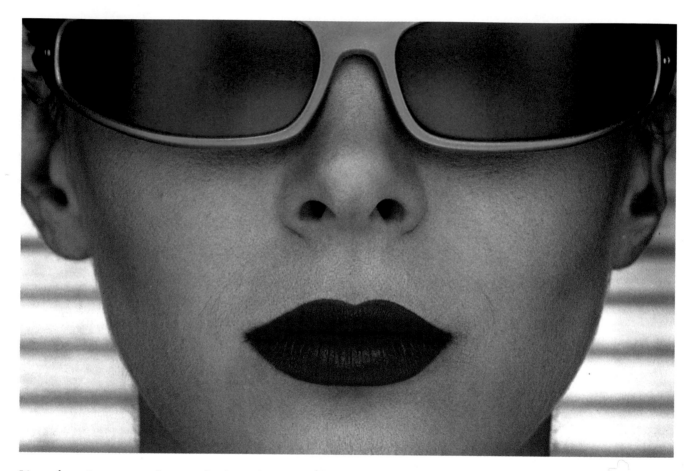

Lip color gives your glamour look its final polish and pizzazz —
which is why you'll want to experiment with different colors, products, and techniques to achieve just the right effect. Lip colors,
glosses, and liners can be mixed and matched for a variety of looks;
in addition, you can use an intensity controller lip color enhancer
to personalize your shade to whatever suits your individual style.

Whether you choose matte or shiny, light or dark, warm or cool,
there's a lip product — and look — to match. Your only guideline:
keeping your lip color and blusher in the same color family, warm
or cool. The rest is up to you. Begin with the color combinations
recommended here; then experiment with choices of your own.

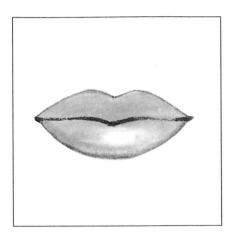

Subtle and Shimmering
For a sheer, natural look, try this technique: begin by applying a thicker line of a light primrose lip-liner pencil along your natural lip line. Next, use a clear lip gloss all over lips, blending the gloss into the pencil to achieve a shiny hint of color. Press lips gently together to blend.

Flirty and Feminine
For irresistible appeal, begin by lining your lips with a medium pink lip-liner pencil. Next, fill in your lips with a rose shade of lip color. The finishing touch — a light pink highlighter shade over your lips to give your mouth a beautifully frosted look.

Rich and Radiant

Two lip colors give this look a special radiance. Begin by lining lips with a berry lip-liner pencil. Next fill in with a warm red lip color. Finally, top with a garnet frost to highlight lips with a touch of color and shine.

Delicate and Delicious

For this lip look, use an intensity controller enhancer under your lip shade for soft, romantic color. To start out, line your lips with a medium pink lip-liner pencil. Next, brush on intensity controller enhancer — again, the more you apply, the lighter your lip color will be. Last, add your lip shade — here, a luscious watermelon. Press lips together to distribute color.

Soft and Sensuous

For barely there color and lots of shine, try this soft and sexy look. First, line lips with a pale pink lip-liner pencil. Next, apply a frosty pink lip color to the outer corners of your lips, leaving the center open. Finally, bring the color together by filling in the center with a light pink lip gloss. Press your lips gently together to blend.

Irresistible and Individual

This simple technique can be adjusted to suit your individual look. Start by lining lips with a medium pink lip-liner pencil. Next, brush on a deep fuchsia lip color. The final step — a neutral intensity controller applied over the fuchsia — the more intensity controller you use, the lighter your lip color will appear.

Putting It All Together

Soft, natural, and country casual are the words that best sum up what Kate requires from a makeup look. She runs a part-time business with her husband from their rural home, and because she deals with customers every day she has to look her best. At the same time, Kate's country setting calls for a natural look that's never overdone. In addition to managing her business Kate is the mother of a toddler and has a fairly tight schedule every day.

Kate chooses a warm color scheme for her glamour makeup — a soft apricot powder blush and a coordinating coral lip color. On her eyes, she uses a wash of cocoa eye shadow accented with cobalt blue eye shadow on the lids. The final touch — navy eye-defining pencil and brown mascara.

The complete look takes only a few minutes each day and is just what Kate needs from her makeup — warm and polished, with a few bright touches that make her best features stand out.

For a look that's soft and polished, Kate keeps her beauty routine simple. In just a few minutes a day, she can achieve the natural, well-groomed appearance her busy lifestyle demands.

June needs a sophisticated daytime look for her career in cosmetics sales. She wants to project an image of glamour and elegance with her daily makeup because she sets beauty standards for the people she works with. June and her husband also entertain frequently, and since she often doesn't have time for more than freshening her daytime makeup in the evening, June needs a makeup look that takes her straight from a busy day into a social evening.

June selects cool cheek and lip shades for her glamour look — a light pink powder blusher on her cheekbones and a slightly deeper shade as a contour; for her lips, medium pink lip-liner pencil and rose lip color. On her eyes she combines several eye shadow shades — shell, plum, and two shades of blue. The colors are blended carefully for a soft yet spectacular effect. To finish the look — a thin line of black eyeliner above and below the lashes and two coats of black mascara.

The complete look offers June the kind of fashionable sophistication she needs for her career and her busy social schedule.

With a career in cosmetic sales and an active social schedule, June needs a makeup look that's sophisticated and long-lasting. She chooses colors and application techniques that take her from day to evening.

Meg has a busy professional city life with an active evening social schedule. She requires makeup that gives her a serious working woman image for day and a sophisticated, elegant style for night.

She chooses a cool glamour look for day — for cheeks, raspberry cream blush followed by violet powder blusher for a long-lasting color; and on her lips, a cool crimson lip color. To accent her eyes, Meg wears a shell highlighter on her brow and a deep plum shadow on the lid. A thin line of black eyeliner and black mascara complete the effect.

A few simple techniques will enhance the look for evening — a touch-up of violet blusher; a clear lip gloss to top her crimson lip color for extra shine; and finally, plum eye shadow and grape eye-defining pencil under her lower lashes to accentuate the color. An extra coat of black mascara and she's ready for a night on the town.

Meg's complete look projects exactly the image she wants to create — for day, the subtle luster of attractive, straightforward makeup; for evening, the touches of glamour that add instant panache. Once she achieves her basic look — the polish of a professional woman — she can quickly convert it to dazzle at the end of her workday.

FOUR

Hair Care

Hair that's everything it should be — soft, shining, healthy, and full of life. Taking care of your hair means keeping it clean and conditioned, choosing a style that complements you and fits in with the details of your beauty program. Your hairstyle — short or long, curly or straight — showcases your features and expresses the importance you place on looking your very best. Because your beautiful hair literally shimmers with health, vitality, and personal style.

Your Hair

Most people take their hair for granted, assuming that if they wash it regularly, it will stay beautiful and healthy. But there's more to beautiful hair than just shampoo and water. To care for your hair properly you should have a basic knowledge of its functions — the factors that contribute to its condition and texture, the amount of hair you have, and its color.

The hair on your scalp is similar to the epidermis, or outer layer, of your skin. Hair is made of dead cells pushed upward by new living cells in the hair follicle. Like the skin's surface, the cells that make up a strand of hair contain the protein keratin. Between one hundred thousand and two hundred thousand hair follicles produce the hair strands on your scalp. Oil (sebaceous) glands attached to the hair follicles produce and secrete the oily substance sebum, which lubricates and smooths the hair strands as they move upward toward the surface.

The average growth rate of hair is approximately one-half inch each month, or six inches a year. After a growing period of four to ten years, the root of each hair goes into a resting period of about three months, during which the base of the hair follicle shrinks and no new cells are produced. At the end of the rest period, hair cells begin to multiply again, pushing new strands of hair toward the scalp's surface and causing the "old" hair to loosen and fall out. As a result it isn't unusual to experience some hair loss daily. (The cycles of growth and rest occur on different schedules all over the scalp so that no one area is losing all its hair at the same time.) Only five thousand to ten thousand hair follicles, scattered over the head, are dormant at any given time.

The texture of your hair is determined by the diameter of each strand of hair. A strand of coarse hair is relatively large in diameter, while a strand of fine hair is relatively small in diameter. If your hair is very thick you probably have a great many hair follicles; if your hair is thin you have a smaller number of hair follicles. The number of hair follicles you have and the size of individual hair strands are basically factors of heredity, although proper conditioning and styling techniques can help correct extremes.

The cross-sectional shape of each strand is what makes hair straight, wavy, or curly: perfectly round strands produce straight hair; flat, oval-shaped hair shafts produce wavy hair; and very curly

A cross section of a strand of growing hair illustrates its structure. Each hair follicle has an arrector pili muscle attached to it. When cold or fear makes the muscles contract, your hair stands straight up and your scalp gets goose bumps.

sebaceous gland

hair shaft

arrector pili muscle

hair follicle

hair is composed of flatter, kidney-shaped strands. This is another genetically determined characteristic of hair.

The color of your hair is governed by melanin, the same pigment that gives color to your skin. Less melanin may be produced as you get older, causing hair to gray.

Your hair can become one of your most versatile and important beauty assets. Whether you wear it long or short, curly or straight, your hair is one of the first things people notice about you. And when you decide to change your cut or style, you know your hair will continue to grow and renew itself constantly. So whatever your preferences in hairstyles, it's essential that you maintain a healthy routine of hair care.

Taking a Closer Look

Every woman wants her hair to be healthy and lustrous, to shine and have lots of bounce. She also wants a flattering hairstyle that is easy to care for. A basic hair-care system lays the groundwork for all these goals. To care for your hair properly, however, you must first understand its characteristics: quantity, type, texture, overall condition, and even the shape and size of each individual hair strand.

The following inventory is designed to help you determine the nature of your hair. Complete the statements below as accurately as possible by evaluating the characteristics of your hair at the present time. If you color your hair, have a permanent, or treat it chemically in any way, circle the appropriate answer with respect to your hair's current condition, rather than its natural state.

The woman at the top has a head of thick hair, whereas the woman in the lower photo is an example of someone with thin hair.

1. **Twenty-four to forty-eight hours after shampooing, regardless of the products I use, my hair:**
   A. Looks and feels better than it does right after shampooing, when it tends to be dull and flyaway.
   B. Does not look or feel significantly different from the way it does right after shampooing.
   C. Feels matted down and greasy; it sticks together in clumps and looks darker at the roots.

2. **My hair generally responds to the cold, dry winter climate and the hot, damp summer climate in the following manner:**
   A. In the winter, my hair becomes very dry and flyaway and often has static electricity; in the summer, my hair seems more stabilized and easier to control.
   B. In the winter, my hair tends to become dry and sometimes has static electricity; in the summer, my hair tends to become slightly oily and limp.
   C. In the winter, my hair seems more normal and I seldom have problems with flyaway hair or static electricity; in the summer, my hair becomes oily and limp and seems to get dirty quickly.

3. **Choose the phrase that most accurately describes the amount and distribution of your hair:**
   A. I have a lot of hair densely distributed over my scalp.
   B. I have a medium amount of hair evenly distributed over my scalp.
   C. I have a less-than-medium amount of hair sparsely distributed over my scalp.

4. **Individual strands of my hair are:**
   A. Large in diameter; my hair has volume and weight.
   B. Of medium size.
   C. Thin and fragile; my hair has little body and tends to be limp.

Answers to statements 1 and 2 generally match. If both answers are *A*, your hair type is dry; if both are *B*, your hair type is normal; and if both are *C*, your hair type is oily. Follow the instructions for your specific hair type throughout this section on hair care and styling.

If one of your answers is *B*, and the other is *A* or *C*, your hair is in the normal range, tending to either dryness or oiliness. Look for the instructions for your hair type tendency, either dry or oily, in the pages that follow.

If you answered *A* and *C* to statements 1 and 2, respectively, your hair condition ranges between the two extreme types, dry to oily. If you answered *C* and *A*, respectively, your hair ranges from oily to dry. These extremes may be caused by cleansing and conditioning products, hair coloring, or other chemical treatments. If you have either type of combination hair, you will probably want to follow the hair-care instructions beginning with the first word in your combination (although you should also consider the season and your lifestyle at the time you begin this care system). Take this inventory again in three months. If your hair falls more into the normal range at that time, adjust your hair care accordingly; if your hair has not improved noticeably, try the hair-care instructions beginning with the second word in your combination type.

If you use coloring agents or treat your hair chemically, take this inventory one week after treating it to note changes in your hair so you can adjust your hair-care routine.

If your answer to statement 3 was *A*, your hair distribution is thick and the quantity large; *B*, medium distribution and medium quantity; *C*, thin distribution and small quantity.

If your answer to statement 4 on hair texture was *A*, you have coarse hair; *B*, medium hair; *C*, fine hair.

The quantity and texture of your hair are not related to its type or condition. Although you can't radically change these characteristics, you can make your hair seem more — or less — full, softer, or coarser by following special hair-care guidelines and selecting appropriate hairstyles.

Record the characteristics of your hair in the spaces provided below. As you read the following pages on hair care and hair styling, refer to this inventory for these characteristics. Look for special considerations for your hair type, texture, distribution, and quantity; these qualities can influence your hair's strength, elasticity, and general appearance.

The hair of the woman at top is coarse in texture; below, the woman's hair is fine in texture.

Hair type _____

Distribution/quantity _____

Texture _____

Discovering Your Hair Type

Your type of hair — dry, normal, or oily — is, like your type of skin, largely determined by heredity. In fact, most people have the same hair and skin types. If your skin is dry, your hair is apt to be dry as well; if you have oily skin, you probably have oily hair. But skin is also affected by the environment in which you live. The oil glands in the area below the scalp have the most influence on the condition of the hair strands themselves. This natural oil is secreted onto the hair shafts in the follicles, and both the amount and distribution of this oil are what determine the dryness or oiliness of your hair.

The water in the tissue below the scalp is responsible for supplying your hair and scalp with its healthful moisture content, which contributes mainly to the elasticity and, somewhat less, to the shine of your hair as well as to the condition of your scalp.

With consistent and proper care, you can make the most of your hair's unique characteristics — and even improve its condition. After taking the personal inventory of hair type on pages 146 and 147, you will be able to identify the special problem of your hair and care for it accordingly.

Dry hair is the result of insufficient oil and moisture in and around the hair shafts. This type of hair is often brittle and breaks easily. While dry hair may seem to grow more slowly, its constant breakage actually prevents it from growing very long. Also, because dry hair tends to fray at the ends, "split ends" can often result. Split ends occur when the cortex of the hair shaft cracks and splits into many tiny fibers. These filamentlike fibers at the shafts' ends catch among other split ends, causing tangling and further breakage when the hair is combed. Regular trimming of split ends should be combined with conditioning to help smooth the cuticles. Moisture and oil are retained on the hair shafts, making them silkier, more slippery, and less likely to tangle.

Bleaching, coloring, and permanent curling of the hair all tend to make it drier and, in some cases, more fragile. If your hair is chemically treated, check the special considerations on pages 154 to 159 to determine the specific care your hair requires.

Normal hair has a proper amount of oil and moisture on the scalp and in and around the hair shafts. Normal hair tends to have good elasticity and shine, with little or no breakage or split ends.

A shaft of your hair is composed of three layers. The cuticle or outer layer is made of hard transparent cells that overlap each other. The cortex or middle layer is composed of protein fibers and is protected by the cuticle. The medulla or center is a partially hollow structure. In some hair shafts, it is normal for the medulla to be absent or interrupted.

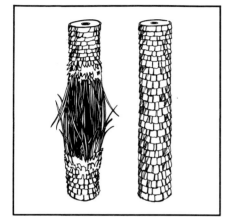

The shine of your hair is determined in part by the condition of the cuticle. When intact, the cuticle's scales form a smooth, even surface that reflects light. When damaged, the scales peel away from the hair shaft; light is not reflected and hair no longer appears shiny and lustrous. A split end — or a mid-shaft split, as shown at left — results from the unraveling of the ropelike fibers of the cortex when the cuticle is damaged.

Regularly cleansing the scalp and hair removes surface soils and helps keep your scalp operating well; moderate conditioning also helps your hair retain its important oil and moisture content. This moisture protects normal hair from the effects of dry environments, as well as from potentially damaging styling techniques such as blow-drying and permanent waving. In general, good hair care helps to maintain normal hair at its beautiful best.

Oily hair tends to be overly lubricated, limp, and lacking in shine as a result of excess oil production from the underlying sebaceous glands. Since both the scalp and the hair become somewhat sticky from the extra oil that coats them, soils stay on the surface of the scalp and hair shafts, contributing to the dull appearance of the hair. You must cleanse oily hair frequently and properly to remove these soils and give your hair added shine. Regular cleansing also helps to control the extra oils on the scalp and hair. Overly oily hair may not require much conditioning, but you may need to use a conditioner occasionally after shampooing to aid you in combing your wet and fragile hair.

Blow-dryers and electric curlers can dry the ends of hair shafts, which are less well supplied with the extra oils produced on the scalp. This results in what appears to be "combination" hair — oily scalp combined with hair that is dry at the ends. If you have combination hair, use conditioners only at the ends of your hair. A good program of hair care can also help normalize oil distribution.

Shampoo

Keeping your hair clean is important to its appearance and to the health of your scalp. Cleansing removes perspiration, soil, and other impurities that stick to your scalp and interfere with its healthful functioning. Shampooing your hair also has obvious beauty benefits: clean hair smells fresh, feels wonderfully silken, and has a lustrous shine and healthy bounce. In order to cleanse your hair properly, you must use the right shampoo for your hair type and condition, and follow the proper procedure for shampooing.

The best shampoos have an acid to neutral-acid pH. Because the surface coating of oils and sweat has an acidic pH, these shampoos are compatible with your hair and leave it clean, soft, smooth, and shiny.

Dry to normal hair needs a gentle cleanser that removes soil without stripping away the oils and moisture that are vital.

Oily hair needs a more active cleanser because the shampoo must remove excess oil and soil from the scalp and hair strands.

How to Shampoo Your Hair Wet your hair and scalp thoroughly with warm water. Pour a small amount of shampoo — a dollop about the size of a quarter — into your palm, then rub your hands together to distribute the shampoo over your palms and fingertips. Don't pour shampoo directly from the bottle onto your hair because you will concentrate it on a single area. Apply the shampoo, working it into a lather with your fingertips. Gently massage your scalp with the balls of your fingers in a circular movement — never scrub with your nails; that could scratch and damage your scalp's delicate surface. Also, never pile your hair on top of your head; instead, allow shampoo and water to run down through your hair. Finish your shampoo by rinsing your hair and scalp thoroughly with clear, warm water, using your fingertips to separate strands of hair. Allow the water to run through your hair for at least thirty seconds to make sure all shampoo is rinsed away.

If your hair is oily, reapply shampoo if necessary following the procedure described above, then rinse again thoroughly for about thirty seconds. For a final rinse — and to harden your hair shafts — let cool water run over your hair and scalp for about ten seconds.

When your hair is thoroughly cleansed, you are ready to apply conditioner.

Thick hair is dense and may tangle easily. Be sure to distribute shampoo gently and evenly, lifting hair up to apply shampoo underneath and on the scalp. Rinse very thoroughly, making sure to remove shampoo from scalp and hair.

Because clean hair appears to have greater volume, shampooing benefits *thin hair* by making it look thicker. Thin hair shafts are fragile, however, so shampoo should be applied very gently and distributed evenly, with as little manipulation of the scalp as possible.

Coarse hair tends to absorb shampoo readily and should be given an extra final rinse to remove all traces of suds.

Fine hair has more body when it's clean, so shampoo it often. Fine hair is very delicate, however, and breaks easily when it's wet. Shampoo gently, using light fingertip movements from scalp to ends.

For best results, work shampoo *gently* into your hair with your fingertips. Then enjoy the fresh exhilaration of a *thorough* rinse — count to thirty as clear water runs over and through your hair. Finally, luxuriate in the clean feel of just-shampooed hair.

Condition

To keep hair shiny and flexible, all types have to be conditioned after shampooing. Natural oils from the scalp coat each strand of hair to give it shine and to seal moisture into the hair shaft. Moisture helps maintain elasticity and strength. Since dry hair does not produce enough natural oil to give the individual strands their protective and beautifying oil coat, a conditioner adds to the natural oil supply and gives dry hair shine as well as bounce and strength. Oily hair, however, may not have sufficient shine because too much oil coats the hair shafts, which are dulled by soil that sticks to them. Shampoos for oily hair remove some of the excess oil while removing soil; a conditioner restores the oil coating on the hair shafts to a normal level.

The best conditioners have an acid pH that is compatible with the scalp's natural acid level. A protein conditioner helps repair damage and strengthen the individual strands of hair. A good conditioner also minimizes tangling by helping smooth the outer layer of each hair shaft with a light coating. An acid pH protein conditioner can give extra body and fullness to oily hair. While protein conditioners are suitable for all types of hair, the method of application is different for each type.

How to Condition Your Hair After shampooing, gently squeeze out excess water from your hair. Pour about one tablespoon of conditioner into your palm and rub your hands together to distribute conditioner over your palms and fingertips. If you have **dry to normal hair**, work the conditioner into your hair, beginning at the ends and distributing it evenly up over the shafts to the roots; if your ends are very dry and/or split, carefully massage extra conditioner into them with your fingertips. Leave the conditioner on your hair for at least one minute, then rinse your hair and scalp thoroughly and gently with clear, warm water for at least sixty seconds. Continue rinsing until all conditioner is removed and your hair feels smooth and slippery, but not greasy.

If you have **oily hair**, begin at your hair ends and work the conditioner gently up the hair strands toward the roots, stopping midway between your hair ends and roots. Avoid getting conditioner on your scalp. Leave the conditioner on your hair for at least one

Keep in Mind . . .

Thick hair benefits from regular conditioning, which reduces its tendency to tangle when it is wet. Distribute conditioner evenly, lifting hair to make sure all of it receives conditioner.

Thin hair may be fragile and pull out easily, so distribute conditioner evenly without handling your hair excessively.

Conditioner helps **coarse hair** by adding extra shine and making it manageable. If your ends tend to fray and split, leave conditioner on ends one minute longer for added conditioning.

Conditioned **fine hair** has more body. Apply conditioner very gently in the direction in which your hair grows. Rinse thoroughly, since conditioner left on fine hair can add to its limpness.

Conditioning adds bounce, softness, and luster to every type of hair. For problem hair, a conditioner is essential after every shampoo. Conditioning smooths the rough outer surface, or cuticle, of damaged strands, and prevents the tangling that can cause further breakage and damage. The photos above show, from left to right, a conditioned hair strand, a split end, and a mid-shaft split.

minute, then rinse thoroughly with warm (not hot) water. Continue rinsing until all conditioner is removed and your hair feels smooth and slippery, but not oily. A final cool-water rinse of your hair and scalp may provide some astringent action and help harden your hair shafts.

How to Dry Your Hair Hair strands are weakest when they are wet and can break or fray easily from hard rubbing with a towel. To prevent tangling and breakage, blot your hair gently with a soft, clean, fluffy towel, pressing gently against your scalp. Then smooth the towel along the length of your hair in the direction in which it grows. Circular or back-and-forth movements tangle your hair, resulting in breakage when you comb out wet hair.

Special Considerations

Regular conditioning after every shampoo can keep your hair healthy. But if your hair becomes seriously damaged, an intensive protein-packed conditioner instead of your regular conditioner can help restore shining flexibility.

Hair becomes dull and loses its bounce when the outer layer, or cuticle, of individual hair strands breaks. Intact, the cuticle's scales make a smooth, even surface that reflects light and gives hair a nice sheen. When the cuticle is damaged, the scales peel away from the hair shaft, preventing light from reflecting evenly and making hair look dull. Once the cuticle is damaged, moisture evaporates from the inner layer of the hair shafts and makes hair brittle, coarse, and dry. Whatever your hair type — dry, normal, or oily — the shafts and ends may become damaged and dry out for many reasons.

Hair can become seriously damaged by regular exposure to excessive sun and/or wind; by home or professional color treatments, including those that lighten or highlight; by permanent waving or curling, chemical relaxing or straightening; or by the use of electric appliances — blow-dryers, curling irons, rollers, hair dryers — several times a week. If you subject your hair to one or more of those appliances, or if your hair is very dry, you should use an intensive conditioner for your specific hair type.

Dry hair should receive an intensive conditioner once a week. After shampooing and lightly towel-drying your hair, apply intensive conditioner from the roots of your hair to the ends of the shafts. Place about one tablespoon of intensive conditioner in your hand, distribute it over your palms and fingertips, and apply it to your hair, working it gently into the strands and distributing it evenly. Leave it on for ten to fifteen minutes; rinse thoroughly.

Normal hair should receive an intensive conditioner twice a month. After shampooing and lightly towel-drying hair, apply intensive conditioner from the roots of your hair to the ends of the shafts, following the same procedure given for dry hair.

Oily hair should receive an intensive conditioner once a month. Apply intensive conditioner to the ends of your hair, working it up the hair shafts to midway between hair roots and ends. (Try not to get intensive conditioner on your scalp.) Leave it on for ten to fifteen minutes. Rinse thoroughly and follow with a cool-water rinse over your hair and scalp.

Keep in Mind . . .

If you wish to increase the manageability of *thick hair,* consider using an intensive conditioner instead of your regular conditioner after every other shampoo. Follow the recommended procedure for your hair type or condition.

Distribute intensive conditioner evenly through *thin hair* without excessively handling your hair or scalp.

Intensive conditioner adds shine and helps prevent *split ends.* Use intensive conditioner after every second shampoo, particularly on your hair ends, following the recommended procedure for your hair type or condition.

Intensive conditioner helps to strengthen and increase the elasticity of *fine hair.* Use intensive conditioner as directed for your hair type.

To protect your hair from the potentially damaging effects of blow-dryers, electric rollers, curling irons, and other appliances, use a protein-packed intensive conditioner regularly.

Combing and Brushing Your Hair

Along with environmental conditions and certain products and appliances, improper combing and brushing can damage your hair.

Comb — never brush — wet hair. (Brushing can snap wet hair shafts when they are most fragile.) Always use a wide-toothed comb with round, smooth teeth that won't snag your hair or scratch your scalp. Comb wet hair from the ends, working out knots and tangles at the bottom of the hair shafts. Lift up segments of hair to work out any tangles underneath. Never pull hard on tangled ends — you'll break individual hair shafts and you may actually pull hair out from its roots. When all the tangles are out, gently run the comb through your hair from the roots down to the ends.

After your hair dries, brushing is beneficial because it helps distribute the natural oils produced in the scalp onto the hair shafts. Brushing can be especially good for *dry to normal hair*, which may not be coated with sufficient oil to keep the hair strands smooth and elastic. If your hair is very *oily*, however, avoid brushing against your scalp. Rather, begin brushing your hair about an inch off your scalp to distribute the oil near your scalp on the ends of hair shafts.

If your hair is *thin*, avoid brushing your scalp. Your hair follicles may be fragile and hair shafts can be pulled out easily.

Fine hair is too delicate and easily broken to withstand much brushing. If your hair is very fine and you need to distribute more oil on your hair shafts, brush very gently and slowly, using a natural bristle brush with widely spaced bristles — or simply comb.

The best brush for all types of hair is one with natural, smooth-ended bristles in well-spaced rows. If your hair seems to catch or snag on the ends of bristles, your brush is probably worn and the bristles frayed or split. This usually means it's time for a new brush.

It's important to keep combs and brushes very clean. About once a week, soak plastic combs and brushes in a solution of one tablespoon of ammonia (or any strong household cleanser) to two quarts of warm water for an hour. For natural bristle brushes use a solution of diluted shampoo. The solutions loosen soil and remove stray hairs trapped on the surfaces of combs and brushes. Rinse combs and brushes thoroughly after soaking and dry them with a clean towel.

Special Considerations

No matter how well you care for your hair, you may discover problems that do not respond to your regular hair-care routine. Difficulties such as dandruff, dry scalp, and hair loss require special treatment. Because many hair and scalp problems may stem from your overall physical condition and be symptoms of a more serious disease, consult your doctor whenever you notice a serious or prolonged change.

Dandruff results in large, loose flakes that accumulate on the scalp and stick to the hair or fall to the shoulders. The disorder is caused by a problem with the reproduction rate of the scalp cells: they multiply much faster than they normally should and reach the surface before they are fully mature. Because the underdeveloped cells have not separated, they flake off in large clumps, rather than as tiny, barely noticeable flakes.

A flake of dandruff, magnified thousands of times.

There is no known preventive treatment for dandruff, and medical experts disagree as to whether the condition is associated with an overly oily or overly dry scalp. Some authorities believe there may be two different types of dandruff, one relating to dryness and one to oiliness.

Nor is there a known cure for dandruff, although there are ways to control it. Compounds such as zinc pyrithione and selenium sulfide, which help scalp cells reproduce at a normal rate, are available in several over-the-counter shampoo formulas. Active compounds such as salicylic acid are also among the ingredients of dandruff shampoos, which help break down and remove scalp cells as they come to the surface.

Dry scalp, as mentioned above, may or may not be a cause of dandruff. Similar to dry skin on any other part of the body, dry scalp may result in minor flaking, not unlike the flaking associated with dry facial skin. You can control dry scalp most effectively by using a very gentle shampoo and an intensive conditioner regularly.

Temporary hair loss can be a result of a number of factors. As new strands of hair form, they loosen and push dormant hair out of the follicles. So it is natural for some of your hair to fall from your scalp during shampooing or brushing. You normally lose about fifty to a hundred strands of hair each day. More than this amount of hair loss could result from any one of a number of factors and may be cause for concern.

Daily repetition of certain hairstyles — especially hair tightly pulled back, braided, or wrapped around rollers — can pull out individual hairs. Over time, such pulling can damage and destroy follicles completely; the hair will not grow back.

Emotional stress may bring on *alopecia areata,* a disorder that results in bald patches on the scalp and may be associated with changes in the immune system. Emotional stress can also cause hair to fall from all parts of the scalp.

Body stress — from high fever or lengthy surgery, for example — is also known to cause excessive hair loss, and evidence exists that medication for high blood pressure and psychological depression can cause hair to shed more rapidly than is normal. In addition, hair loss can result from pregnancy (it usually appears after delivery) or begin when a woman stops taking birth control pills. Hormonal changes that occur during pregnancy and while using birth control pills cause more hair follicles to remain dormant. After a woman gives birth, or when she discontinues using birth control pills, the renewal growth cycle begins, and the "old" hairs are pushed out and shed by the new growth. This cycle can continue for up to six months following pregnancy and delivery. Some women also notice that their hair becomes much drier during pregnancy. The condition is best controlled by using a very gentle shampoo and an intensive conditioner — instead of a regular conditioner — as often as after every other shampoo.

Most hair loss is temporary, but when the follicles are destroyed by serious scalp burns, excessive exposure to x-rays, or viral infection, hair loss can be permanent.

Special Considerations

The natural color of your hair is determined by the same pigments that determine the tone of your skin. As we grow older, the pigment-producing melanocyte cells may produce less, resulting in graying of the hair.

Your age at the time your hair begins to turn gray is largely a factor of heredity, as are all aspects of your natural hair color. When hair turns gray, it also may become dry, generally because the amount of oil produced in the scalp decreases as we get older. Increased use of an intensive conditioner can benefit dry hair, as can the use of a gentle shampoo for dry to normal hair.

Premature graying is an inherited characteristic; it may or may not be accompanied by dry hair. If your family history includes early graying, your hair could gray at almost any point in your life, sometimes as early as your late teens.

Gray hair can be very attractive, but if you prefer not to have gray hair or wish to change your hair color for any reason, many coloring options are available to you.

Chemical treatments for hair — including single- and double-process hair color, straightening or relaxing curly hair, and permanent waving — alter the structure of the inner layer of hair shafts. The chemicals lift up and penetrate the outer layer. As a result, hair may appear drier, more brittle, or less vital than before treatment because the scales that form this outer layer are damaged and do not reflect light evenly.

The physical effect of chemical treatments also causes individual strands of hair to increase in diameter and become more porous, especially at the ends. If your hair is thin and/or fine in texture, chemical treatments can add desirable body to your hair by expanding the shafts, making your hair look thicker and coarser. If your hair is very thin, fine, and fragile, however, strong chemical treatments may weaken it further, causing breakage. If you are not sure how fragile your hair is, ask a professional hairdresser how well the distribution and texture of your hair will react to chemical treatments.

Hair coloring agents such as henna, which coat your hair shafts without changing their outer layer, are another coloring option. Henna can deepen brown and black hair and add reddish highlights to all colors of hair. Henna tends to protect the hair's cuticle and

Hair changes with age, and the most obvious change is graying. Many women like the look of healthy, well-styled, and well-cared-for gray hair. Simple treatments, however, provide color options for those who want an alternative to gray.

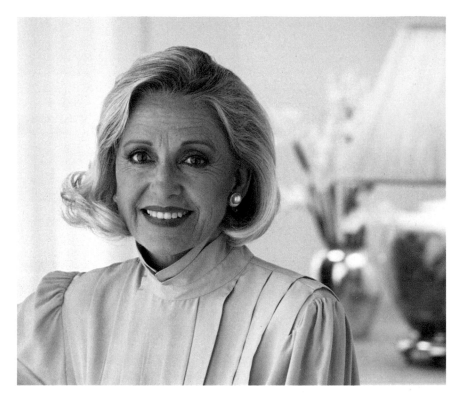

makes hair appear thicker and glossier. Neutral hennas add no color, but still make thin and/or fine hair appear to be thicker and have more body. Henna does not take well, however, on blond or gray or coarse hair, all of which absorb too much color and may be dulled by the henna colorants.

Conditioners applied immediately after chemical treatment help smooth the cuticle layer so hair becomes shinier and more flexible. Conditioners can help prevent hair that has been colored with a double-process method, or colored and permanent-waved, from breaking.

Some chemicals used in hair coloring, waving, or straightening formulas irritate the scalp. To prevent irritation or allergic reactions, professional beauticians often apply a protective cream to the scalp before applying the chemicals to the hair shafts themselves. If your scalp is sensitive, ask your hairdresser to use a cream before your chemical treatments.

Coloring and permanent waving products designed for at-home use are generally not as strong as those used by professionals. As a result, protecting your scalp may not be necessary, but it is still a good idea to keep the treatment on your hair and away from your scalp. Always check first for a possible allergic reaction by patch-testing according to instructions on the package.

our Hairstyle

On pages 160 to 163 we'll look at what role the shape of your face and various style elements play in choosing a hairstyle. But your lifestyle is a major determinant. If you wash, condition, and style your hair every morning, a short haircut may be best for you because it takes less time to care for. If you exercise three times a week or more, you may find short hair more manageable and easier to keep clean than long hair.

If you have plenty of time for hair care and find that your hair holds a flattering style for several days at a time, you may prefer to wear your hair long — pulled back from your face in a tidy knot for business days or styled in lavish curls for special nights out.

The distribution and quantity of your hair also play a part in your choice of hairstyle. Short or layered cuts make thick hair more manageable. A blunt cut adds thickness to thin hair, especially if you wear it medium length to your chin. Very short cuts and very long cuts can make thin hair look thinner, unless you add volume with curl.

The texture of your hair is another factor in selecting a style. Coarse hair often looks best short or, when worn long, thinned or layered. Because coarse hair holds curls and waves very well, it keeps a style longer than other types do and may not require too much styling time if you wear it long. Fine hair needs the body it gets from styles worn shoulder length or shorter. Longer styles tend to make fine hair look limp and shapeless, but permanent waves add both volume and body.

The curliness or straightness of your hair should also be considered in your hairstyle choices. Very curly hair is easiest to manage when worn short. Wavy hair has a tendency to become curlier when it is short, and to become straighter as it grows. Straight and difficult-to-curl hair is best worn in simple styles — well-shaped short cuts, medium-length blunt cuts, or longer styles that can be pulled back, worn up in a knot or bun, or dressed up with accessories (see page 163).

Finally, your height should influence your choice of hairstyle. If you're tall, very short styles can make your face seem proportionately small; medium to longer lengths, worn full, offer better balance to a tall frame. If, in addition, you have a long neck, styles with greater length at the back are best. If you're short, long hairstyles tend to exaggerate your lack of height.

Longer hair is very versatile: you can wear it up for a sleek, sophisticated look or down for one that's full and feminine. Short hair is pert, pretty, and stylish; it's easy to care for and perfect for today's more active lifestyles.

How you wear your hair — long, short, straight, curly, or wavy — will depend on your hair's natural characteristics and your own personal needs and preferences. The hairstyle that's right for you makes the most of your hair's best qualities.

Talking to Your Hairdresser

Here are tips on telling your hairdresser what look you want.

Think about what you want your hairstyle to do for you and explain it carefully to your hairdresser. Take along a picture of the style you want to try, but be sure it is appropriate for your hair type and face shape.

Listen to your hairdresser and have confidence in his or her opinions once you've found someone you like.

Speak up about the qualities of your hair. Does it hold curl well? Does it need extra body, shine, volume, a brighter color? Also, tell your stylist a little bit about yourself and your lifestyle: Do you have only ten minutes in the morning to style your hair? Can you handle a blow-dryer easily? Are your requirements different for work and play?

Be courteous. Book your appointments well in advance and, if you must cancel, give at least twenty-four hours' notice. And be punctual!

Be honest. If you don't like the work your hairdresser has done, tell the stylist why, as tactfully as you can. In many cases, the problem can be corrected before you leave the salon. And if you love what a hairdresser has done, tell that to him or her too! (A tip of 15 to 20 percent, except for a salon owner, also expresses your appreciation.)

Your Hairstyle

The way you wear your hair — parted, pulled back, with or without bangs — can affect the appearance of your features, highlighting and dramatizing them. Your personal style will always be a factor in the hairstyles you choose. Long styles and curls add softness and femininity. Short, straight hair has elegance and style. Hair worn back from your face and up off your neck is dressed-up and dramatic. Braids and ponytails are youthful and winsome. Very curly hair has a lively, spirited look. Wavy hair looks rich and distinctive.

Because hair-care technology offers so many options, you can make your hair look almost any way you want it to. Curly hair can be straightened and straight hair can be curled. Drab hair can be brightened, and unexciting hair colors can be lightened, darkened, or highlighted. Thin or fine hair can acquire more volume and body through special care and styling. Coarse or thick hair can be tamed and made softer and smoother by proper hair care and hair-cuts. Long hair can be cut shorter and short hair can be allowed to grow. What's most exciting about your hair is that there are so many possibilities to choose from.

To maximize the health and beauty of your hair, always start with a basic hair-care system designed for your hair type or condition. You can find one style you love and stay with it — or you can change your hair with the seasons, and experiment with color, length, style, curl, or wave. On the following pages, we show you how to put together all you've learned about hair care and style and make it yours.

Bangs worn straight across your forehead make your brow seem wider and draw attention to your eyes. Bangs that are long at the temples and curve up to a shorter length across your forehead also emphasize your eyes and make cheekbones look broader. Curly or wavy bangs soften angles on your upper face. The length of your bangs influences the appearance of your forehead: short bangs make the distance between eyebrows and hairline look longer than it is; long bangs make your forehead look shorter and sometimes wider.

Parts worn straight down the center add width to your brow, but may emphasize a long nose. Slightly off-center parts and side parts make your forehead seem narrower and can shorten the appearance of a long nose. Low side parts on your head broaden your forehead and help detract from your nose.

Hair pulled straight back or up off your neck draws attention to your facial shape. This style highlights your jawline, elongates and thins your neck, and can make your ears appear larger than they are. Drawing your hair over the tops of your ears when you wear it back from your face helps make your ears look smaller and closer to your head. Hair worn away from your face can also accentuate a small or large nose, an effect that can be diminished by wearing bangs across your forehead when you wear your hair back or up.

166

Fullness at the crown tends to make your face look longer; at your temples, fullness adds width to your cheeks and brow; and fullness at your jawline or below broadens your lower face. Waves or curls worn in styles that come in close on your face tend to make it look narrower; full hair brushed up and away from your face at your temples gives a lift to your cheekbones and makes your eyes look wider.

Tendrils — wisps of wavy or curly hair that fall from a pulled-up hairstyle — soften the outer edge of your face and add length to your neck. Tendrils can soften the severity of a hairstyle pulled back from your face.

Pretty Accessories for Your Hair

No matter what hair length or style you choose, accessories can add interest, color, and extra hold. **Barrettes** or **combs** capture stray hairs, hold hair away from your face, or flatten your hair. Or use combs to sweep hair up and back at your temples to give your whole face a lift. For easy height at your crown, push a comb upward at the top of your head. Select combs with round or softly pointed teeth and no sharp edges to snag or tangle hair. **Headbands,** and scarves or ribbons used as headbands, are great for taming hair that has too much volume, or for holding hair when you're exercising. **Flowers** can be fastened in your hair almost anywhere. Cut the stems of fresh flowers to no more than two inches and secure them with bobby pins. If you like, glue a **ribbon** or **bow** onto a plain barrette, comb, or headband. Or tie ribbons around ponytails and braids to disguise covered elastics (plain rubber bands can break your hair).

Taking a Closer Look

Use your hairstyle as a beauty accessory to complement those features of your face you wish to highlight, and to draw attention away from the features you wish to camouflage. Check the inventories on pages 92 to 95 to recall the aspects of your face you would like to enhance and those you are more interested in playing down. Then look for your basic facial shape in the drawings on these pages to find the most flattering hairstyle for you.

A *round face* benefits from a hairstyle that adds angles and helps conceal broad, round cheeks. Short hair should be at least as long as the bottoms of your earlobes, with most of your hair at the top and less on the sides, where your hair should be brought toward your face. Long hair should be worn with curls or waves surrounding your face, with most of your hair near your jaw, neck, or shoulders. Hair pulled straight back, worn in bangs, or cropped closely around the temples and cheeks accentuates roundness.

A *square jaw and brow* are best softened by a curly or wavy hairstyle that rounds off the angles of your face. Full, all-over curls should be at least as long as your jaw to detract from the squareness of your lower face. Off-center or swept-to-the-side bangs in soft curls or waves soften the wide angles of your brow. Curls or waves should be worn forward on the outer edges of your face from your forehead to your jawline to further soften your face. Straight hair worn in a blunt cut with straight bangs emphasizes hard-edged angles and can give your face an unbecoming geometrical flatness.

An ***oval face*** can be enhanced by a variety of simple hairstyles. Clean lines highlight this facial shape best; whether long or short, your hairstyle will be most flattering if you wear it straight or slightly wavy. Short styles look best worn away from your face, with most of your hair near your crown. Long hair is most flattering to an oval face when brushed or held back from your face. Or to break the regular lines of an oval face, wear your hair in a side ponytail at the nape of your neck or in an off-center knot near your crown. Few styles detract from the pleasant curves of an oval face, but hair worn very full at the sides can make your face appear too narrow and long. Hairstyles should be in proportion to the width of your face.

A ***triangular face*** can have a narrow jaw and wide cheeks and brow. The best hairstyles for this shape face are those worn close to your head, away from your face at your forehead and temples, with hair fuller from eye to chin level. If your hair is all one length, wear it pulled back at the top and softly waved or curled around your jawline. Or add weight and width to your lower face with a layered cut cropped short around your forehead and temples, and left full around your jaw, neck, and shoulders. Hair cut shorter than the bottoms of your earlobes and close to your face emphasizes wide cheeks and brow, diminishing a narrow jaw and small chin.

Another common ***triangular face*** has a broad jaw and narrow cheeks and brow. This face looks best with hairstyles worn full at your temples, with straight or waved bangs across the width of your forehead. A center or low side part also adds width to your brow. The best styles are short, at earlobe level or above, to bring the eye upward, away from your full jawline. Hairstyles that are straight or pulled back from your forehead and temples, and that fall at your jaw, exaggerate the greater width of your lower face and emphasize cheekbones that are too close together.

Putting It All Together

Karen has a part-time job that keeps her busy when she's not taking care of her home and family. She needs simplicity and ease from a hairstyle — her life is busy and she has to schedule hair care into a week that includes at least three exercise classes. For this reason, Karen keeps her style straight and simple and concentrates on regular trims every two months to control split ends and keep her cut well shaped.

Karen's hair type is normal, but it tends to get dirty easily because she exercises frequently. She finds her shower after each activity a good time to wash and condition her hair. She uses an intensive conditioner on the lower half of her hair strands twice a month after shampooing.

Karen has a medium quantity of hair that is very straight and difficult to curl. Her hair is also coarse to medium in texture and doesn't take permanents and sets evenly. For Karen, a blunt cut, at chin level, offers shape and style without requiring waves and curl. It also makes her hair look fuller and thicker than it actually is.

When she exercises, Karen ties her hair back in a ponytail and uses a headband under her bangs. For elegant evenings, she pulls back her hair in a braided twist at the nape of her neck, holding the sides with barrettes or fastening a flower next to the twist. Sometimes, for important days at work, she adds an off-center topknot, fastening the short stray ends at the sides and back with decorative combs.

Karen's hair care and styling center around her lifestyle and the characteristics of her hair. With straight, hard-to-curl, somewhat coarse hair, she relies on an excellent haircut to give her the shape and style she needs. She uses an intensive conditioner and has her hair trimmed regularly to help her split-ends problem. The length of her hair allows her to pull it up and off her face during strenuous activity, as well as dress up her hairstyle for special occasions. Good basic hair care keeps Karen's hair shiny, manageable, and soft; simple styling accentuates the natural qualities of her hair.

Putting It All Together

Janice needs a feminine and stylish look for her job and prefers the versatility of a long hairstyle. Her lifestyle also allows her enough time in the evenings to care for her shoulder-length blond hair.

Janice's hair is in the normal to dry range and doesn't need daily washing and conditioning. Because of its length, her hair requires time for proper washing and conditioning, so she sets aside two or three evenings a week for this purpose. She uses regular conditioner on her hair after every shampoo and applies an intensive conditioner after every third or fourth shampoo.

Her thick hair demands little special care. She finds that nightly brushing adds shine and helps distribute the oils from her scalp on the hair shafts. She takes extra care in combing her hair when it's wet because it tends to tangle easily.

Janice's medium-textured hair holds styles well because it's thick. Her hairdresser brightens its color with professional highlighting about once every three months, giving her hair a subtle lift of color. The highlighter makes her hair appear dry, so she makes sure she uses an intensive conditioner regularly.

Janice gets regular trims about four times a year (when she has her hair highlighted), and finds that her hair holds its shape nicely when she allows it to dry naturally. For casual weekends, she doesn't have to style it at all. But for the polished look she needs for her career, Janice uses a curling iron on mornings, after she's shampooed and conditioned, to add a fashionable upswept look to her style. After her hair is dry she sometimes lifts the side segments of hair to curl them up and back with the curling iron. Since her hair holds curl well, she only has to touch up the style occasionally between shampoos.

Janice helps maintain her strong, healthy hair with a basic hair-care system, taking the time to use an intensive conditioner regularly to counteract the drying effects the curling iron and the highlighting color treatments have on her hair. For casual days, she may braid her hair and tie the ends with pretty ribbons; for elegant evenings, she often wears her hair down and pulled behind her ears, giving her a youthful but stylish look.

Putting It All Together

Daily shampooing and proper home and professional care keep Maryanne's hair shiny and soft. A good hair stylist gives Maryanne the style, shape, and color she wants, and the right hair-care system helps maintain her hair's healthy vitality and bounce.

Maryanne is a successful working mother who doesn't have much time for hair styling before she goes off to work. She wants her hair to look great all the time with as little care as possible.

Maryanne's oily hair needs frequent washing. Since it looks best right after shampooing, she finds it easiest and most beneficial to wash her hair every morning in the shower.

Because her hair is thin and she needs an easy-to-care-for style that will work for her every day, Maryanne keeps her hair short and permed. She conditions it daily to give her hair extra body and shine; once a month, she uses an intensive conditioner on the ends, which dry out from the permanent.

Maryanne consulted her hairdresser about ways to increase the body of her hair and improve its color. Because she usually gives herself home permanents for curl, and the chemicals can affect the hair color, she wanted a professional opinion on adding color. Her stylist didn't want to use a strong peroxide-based coloring agent on Maryanne's permed hair, so he suggested a deep auburn henna. The henna brightens Maryanne's natural coloring, while adding shine, body, and pretty highlights to her hair. She has her hair colored about every eight weeks, when she has it trimmed.

Maryanne finds she can style her hair quickly after her morning shampoo and conditioning. She carefully dries and combs through her hair, then fluffs it up with her fingertips. By the time she's put on her makeup, made breakfast for the baby, and dressed for work, her hair is dry and she's ready to leave for the office. For dressy occasions, Maryanne adds a flower-adorned barrette over one ear.

FIVE

Body Care

Smooth, glowing body skin reflects the care and attention you give your body. By giving top priority to your health and well-being; getting enough sleep and exercise; taking time to relax; and finally, expressing your mood and personality through clothing and fragrance to create your unique sense of style, you show your concern for making your body its beautiful best.

our Body's Skin

The skin on your body is similar to that on your face in basic structure. But greater and lesser distribution of glands and tissues all over your body makes body skin function differently. You can clearly observe that the skin on your eyelids is quite different from the skin on the palms of your hands or the skin on your shoulders. Texture, hair growth, the presence of sebaceous (oil) and sweat glands, nerve endings, and amounts of fat and muscle vary widely over your entire body.

A good example of this variance is the distribution of oil glands that lubricate the surface of the skin. They are most prevalent in the skin of the face, scalp, and upper trunk, while no equivalent glands exist in the palms of hands or soles of feet. Similarly, sweat glands called the apocrine glands are almost exclusive to the underarms and genitals. These glands secrete a milky substance that, when broken down by bacteria on the skin's surface, produces the characteristic odor of human perspiration. The more common sweat glands, the eccrine glands, are far more numerous on the body. The palms of the hands, soles of the feet, and armpits contain the greatest number of eccrine glands; the head, trunk, and limbs have the next highest concentration.

The hands and feet are unique in that they produce fingernails and toenails, which are made of keratin, the same protein found in the epidermis and hair. In nails, keratin forms a thick, translucent plate, strengthening and protecting fingers and toes. The pale half-moon at the bottom of each nail is the root where cells push upward to form the hard nail. The cuticle — the small, somewhat tough fold of skin at the bottom of the nail — protects the area where new cells grow. Nails grow about one-tenth of one millimeter each day, and it takes six months for a nail to replace itself.

Some parts of the body are more sensitive to touch than others because of the kinds and distribution of nerve cells in the lower layers of body skin. Nerve fibers vary in thickness and sensitivity; thin nerve fibers may transport signals, or impulses, more slowly to the nervous system and the brain than do thick ones. In addition, when nerve receptors are close together — as on the fingertips and lips — they are more sensitive. When these fibers are farther apart — as on the backs of the hands — the skin may be less responsive to touch.

Skin, your largest organ, functions differently in various areas of your body. The skin covering your fingertips and lips, for example, is highly sensitive to touch; the soles of your feet contain a large concentration of sweat glands; the perspiration secreted by your underarms is different from that of most other parts of your body. The distinct nature of your body skin requires a beauty-care routine suited to its specific characteristics, functions, and needs.

our Body's Skin

Both facial and body skin are highly vulnerable to the damaging effects of the sun and need protection from ultraviolet radiation (see pages 73 and 194 and 195). The drying effects of the sun can be particularly harmful to your entire torso and arms and legs because this skin contains fewer sebaceous glands.

The skin on your body needs as much careful health and beauty attention as does the skin on your face. But because your body skin functions differently from your facial skin, your body skin-care routine needs to vary from the regimen for your face. For more specific differences between body and facial skin, refer to the chart on the opposite page.

Your Skin from Head to Toe

Factors	Facial Skin	Body Skin
Aging	Your face is constantly exposed to the environment, including the sun and other factors that increase its potential for rapid aging.	You generally cover and protect your body skin with clothing, reducing the drying effects of the environment.
Oiliness	Many large sebaceous glands in the dermis provide skin with more surface oils.	Fewer and smaller sebaceous glands in the dermal layer tend to make skin dry.
Fat	The fatty layer and the dermis are thin, providing less protection from temperature changes and physical trauma.	The fatty layer is thick, in general, and may be very dense in certain areas of the body. Combined with a generally thick dermis, this adds greater support to surface skin and insulation to the body.
Wrinkles	Muscles attached to skin layers are directly involved with the skin's movement. The frequent use of these many small muscles eventually results in lines forming on the surface skin. Also, more sun exposure means more wrinkles.	Muscles attached to underlying joints and bones may be quite large. Since large areas of the body move together, wrinkling tends to be minimal. Also, less sun exposure means fewer wrinkles.
Sensitivity	Nerve endings are close together, so receptivity to stimulation is greater.	Nerve endings are farther apart (except in the fingertips), resulting in reduced sensitivity to outside stimuli.

Special Considerations

The skin that covers your body is a highly efficient organ that, with proper care, will stay healthy. Nonetheless, some conditions of body skin will not respond to even the most careful skin-care routine, and may require medical care.

Psoriasis can appear on any part of the body, although it most often develops on scalp, knees, and elbows. It is characterized by patches, called plaques, of scaly, shedding skin that vary in size and range in color from red to white to silvery. Normal skin cells harden, die, and are shed singly off when they reach the outer layer of the skin's surface. In psoriasis, however, the production of new cells below is too swift, and the surface skin begins to shed large clumps of cells that are not completely hardened to make room for the new cells. It is estimated that psoriasis affects 2 percent of the American population. The condition is not contagious and, while it cannot be cured, it can be controlled in most instances through medical treatment by a dermatologist.

Eczema can cover a wide range of skin problems. One of these, medically known as *atopic dermatitis*, seems to be related to an extreme susceptibility to some form of irritation or is caused by an allergic reaction. Skin affected by eczema becomes dry, scaly, red, and very itchy, most often where the skin is sensitive, as on the insides of elbows and backs of knees. Atopic eczema is believed to be hereditary and may be associated with other disorders, such as asthma, hay fever, and conjuctivitis. The atopic eczema victim may also have a number of allergies and be supersensitive to soaps and detergents.

Prickly heat is known medically as *miliaria*. One form, *miliaria rubra*, results when underlying sweat glands become blocked, usually after prolonged exposure to hot, humid conditions. It is aggravated by the pressure of tight or binding clothing at the waist, shoulders, buttocks, and thighs, which does not allow perspiration to evaporate readily. Affected areas become red, irritated, and extremely itchy, sometimes producing a rash of small red dots. Prickly heat can usually be relieved by seeking a cooler, drier environment and wearing clothing that does not press against the skin.

Scarring results in a visible patch of new skin, different from the surrounding skin, and is usually due to damage which occurs over a large or deep area. Because the skin is constantly regenerating new

Athlete's Foot

Healthy human skin is populated with microorganisms that are usually harmless. However, the fungi that cause athlete's foot tend to multiply and cause an itchy, irritated rash between the toes and in the small crevices of the feet. While this fungus is always present on the skin, it can multiply rapidly in damp areas of skin. The result is the uncomfortable condition called athlete's foot, which is very contagious. The best precaution is to keep your feet clean and dry, particularly after they have been on surfaces where the fungi may have been deposited by others (locker rooms, showers). Over-the-counter topical ointments and powders can help clear up athlete's foot, but in severe cases, a physician should be consulted.

cells, superficial cuts and abrasions are usually repaired rather quickly. In damage extending deeper than the epidermis, blood rushes to fill the cut area. This blood hardens into a clot that attaches itself to the sides of the cut and protects the new connective tissue and epidermis being produced from the surrounding skin. This tissue grows below the clot, filling in the space that remains while the clot shrinks. Depending on the amount of repairs necessary, this might be noticeable as a scar.

Getting immediate medical attention for large cuts in the skin is the best way to prevent scarring. Treatments can close the cut skin and reduce the size of a scar. Once scars have formed, the most effective way to conceal them is cosmetically, by use of an opaque, masking foundation product. Scars that cover a large area on a highly visible part of the body and whose appearance is very disturbing may be improved through surgical techniques.

First-degree **burns** are the least serious, primarily affecting the upper layers of skin and resulting in redness from dilated blood vessels near the skin's surface. Second-degree burns produce blistering and the accumulation of fluid between the dermis and epidermis. In third-degree burns, both the epidermal and part of the dermal layers of skin in the affected area are destroyed, leaving the underlying tissue vulnerable to infection. Such burns are treated, in most cases, by skin grafting, a surgical process in which skin from another part of the body is removed to cover the area that has lost its skin. The transplanted skin adapts to the new area and grows out from its edges to form a new covering. The site from which the skin patch was taken simply regenerates skin cells to provide a new skin surface.

Taking a Closer Look

Your body is affected by the way you live — how much exercise and sleep you get, how well you eat, how healthy you are, and how much attention you pay to yourself, like caring for your skin, hands, and feet. Just as your skin, makeup, and hair project the message that you feel good about yourself, so does the way you take care of your body. You'll want to do everything you can to keep your body toned and fit. The following inventory will guide you in evaluating your needs and goals.

1. **My usual day is:**
   A. Very active; I'm out and about, on my feet, and moving a lot.
   B. Mostly sedentary; I sit at a desk or other work station all day.
   C. A combination of active and sedentary.

2. **I usually have the most leisure time:**
   A. In the morning.
   B. At midday or in the afternoon.
   C. In the evening.
   D. On weekends.

3. **My favorite kind of exercise is:**
   A. Competitive sports (one on one or team games).
   B. Noncompetitive sports where I can improve at my own pace.
   C. Walking or other less strenuous activities.

4. **I sleep well at night and get plenty of rest:**
   A. Usually.
   B. Sometimes.
   C. Seldom.

5. **The area where I live is:**
   A. Urban.
   B. Suburban.
   C. Rural.

6. **The climate in my area (check all that apply):**
   A. Changes with the seasons in temperature and humidity.
   B. Is mostly humid.
   C. Is mostly dry.
   D. Remains quite cold.
   E. Remains hot and sunny.

7. **I would like to improve the way I take care of my:**
   A. Body skin.
   B. Hands and feet.
   C. Figure.

There are many forms of relaxation and exercise, and it is important to make time for all of them. Outdoor activities are necessary for your overall beauty and health.

Statement 1: Because fitness is one of today's beauty essentials, it's important to include some activity in your daily schedule. Where, when, how, and with whom you exercise depends on your personal preferences and needs; the key is making the commitment to stick with the regular program. If you work in an office, it's especially important to make exercise a priority in your day. Still, no matter what kind of work you do, you'll most likely find that exercise is an excellent way to refresh, relax, and unwind.

Statements 2 and 3: For optimum results, tailor your shape-up to fit your lifestyle. Determine what time is best for you — morning, midday, or evening — and select an appropriate activity. Whether you choose an early jog, a brisk lunchtime walk, or an evening tennis match, you'll want to plan ahead. Look closely at your schedule and know your limitations. If you need more discipline, sign up for a class or pre-book court time. Exercise with a friend or join group activities. Whatever you choose, make it something you enjoy. If you look forward to your exercise time — if you equate fitness with fun — the more likely it is your efforts will be successful.

Statement 4: Along with regular exercise, getting enough sleep is important to looking and feeling your best. The information on pages 204 and 205 addresses the need for proper sleep and relaxation. What you want to remember is that when you feel good —

when you've gotten enough sleep, you've taken time to relax, and you've included exercise in your day — you'll be more productive in everything you do.

Statements 5, 6, and 7: Along with staying fit, you want to keep your body skin in tiptop shape. No matter where you live — in the city, the suburbs, or the country — you need to protect your skin from the harmful effects of the sun. Included in the body-care section are tips for giving your body the protection it needs. Another big consideration is the climate you live in; pages 66 and 67 explain how to care for and protect your skin in all types of weather.

A beautiful body — fit, trim, smooth, soft, and well groomed — is an attainable goal. Make it yours with the direction, motivation, and effort offered on the following pages.

Body Skin Care

For body skin that glows with healthy radiance, you need to follow an effective, ongoing skin-care routine. Because its structure is different from that of facial skin, and because much of it is less exposed to the environment, body skin has somewhat different needs. Total body care begins with a basic four-step program that leaves you feeling wonderfully rejuvenated all over: softly polished shoulders, sleek, smooth arms and legs, beautiful hands, and pretty feet.

This scientifically based and uniquely balanced program to care for and beautify your body skin is based on these four simple steps: cleanse, buff, moisturize, and protect. When followed regularly, these steps will give you the beautiful body skin you want — clean, silky smooth, and glowing. Your body-care routine should feel refreshing, help your skin perform at its best, and leave your skin looking radiant and healthy.

Cleanse
Begin by gently washing away the daily buildup of surface dirt, oils, and impurities on your skin, using a rich gel that gently foams away soils while helping to soften the skin and maintain its natural acid balance. Proper cleansing should leave your skin feeling fresh and clean, not tight and dry.

Buff ▲

After cleansing gently, use a buffing cream with a mild abrasive to whisk away dead surface cells, smooth rough calluses on heels, knees, hands, and elbows, and give a smooth, polished finish to your shoulders, arms, and legs. Like a facial mask for your body, buffing stimulates, smooths, and softens.

Moisturize ▶

After you have cleansed and buffed, apply a rich, creamy moisturizer to your shoulders, arms, torso, hips, buttocks, and legs — everywhere. Moisturizer helps lock in surface moisture, leaving skin soft and silky. It should not leave a greasy after-feel.

Protect

Beautifully cleansed, buffed, and moisturized skin needs protection from the sun to maintain its youthful softness and glow. A sunscreening lotion with a sun protection factor of at least 10 guards your body skin against harmful ultraviolet rays and helps prevent the premature aging and dehydration caused by exposure to the sun.

Cleanse

A regular cleansing routine is important to the overall health and glow of your skin. Perspiration from your body's sweat glands can be broken down by the normal bacteria present on your skin's surface to produce an unpleasant odor. Regular cleansing prevents perspiration and bacteria from accumulating.

Cleansing must be effective enough to get your skin really clean and, at the same time, gentle enough to help your skin retain its natural lubrication. A body cleansing gel gently foams away surface soils, perspiration, and bacteria without irritating or drying the surface of the skin. The rich foam also feels wonderful and rinses off easily, leaving the skin clean, silky, and refreshed.

How and When to Cleanse In the shower or bath, squeeze body cleansing gel on your wet hands and lather your entire body until you have worked up a rich foam. To help stimulate your skin and loosen dead surface cells, apply the gel to a body brush, natural bath sponge, or washcloth and gently scrub your body. (If your back is acne-prone or tends to break out, do not use an abrasive on it as this may further irritate the condition. A soft sponge is best for any area of the body that is easily irritated.)

As you cleanse, pay special attention to areas that have the greatest number of sweat glands and therefore tend to produce odors — the underarms, groin, and feet. When you use cleansing gel in your bath, pour it under the running water, as you would bubble bath, to get lots of rich suds. Lather your body well with the suds and put a bit more gel on your applicator to work up extra foam all over. Be sure to rinse well to remove all traces of lather. For a final rinse, take a quick shower.

What time of day you bathe is a matter of personal preference, but bear in mind that your body's sweat glands are active throughout the day, even in cold weather, because perspiration is activated by emotions as well as by the temperature. Cleansing is the first vital step in total body care. Keeping your skin clean makes it look attractive and function beautifully. The soft, silky feeling and fresh, light scent of just-washed skin will give you extra confidence all day long. Proper cleansing is the basis of your body skin care — the groundwork for the next important steps to follow.

Cleansing, your first step in body care, can be as good for your spirits as it is for your skin. Morning showers wake you up and help you start your day refreshed. Evening showers revitalize your spirits and help you go from day to evening. A bath before bed is relaxing and soothing, allowing you to slip between the sheets feeling wonderfully clean. In the bath or shower, a gently foaming body cleansing gel makes your skin feel baby soft, smooth and silky, and totally clean.

Buff

Your body skin, like your facial skin, is constantly renewing itself. As new skin cells are produced and move upward to form the top layer of the skin, they harden and die off to form the protective surface of the skin. Older cells separate from the skin's surface in tiny flakes or build up as a callus. To keep your skin clear and glowing and functioning properly, calluses should be removed.

Buffing body skin aids its natural cell-sloughing process (which tends to slow down with age) and leaves a fresh skin surface. Buffing also helps remove hard patches or calluses that form on elbows, knees, hands, or feet. Because the newly exposed skin must also be guarded against excessive loss of moisture, your buffing product should have a mild cream base. Extra-fine buffing grains in a rich formula help remove the dead cells that can dull the skin's natural glow. Buffing cream leaves your skin brighter, more translucent, and satiny to the touch.

How and When to Buff It's best to use buffing cream twice a week, or about every three days, immediately after washing with cleansing gel. Apply the cream to your fingers and spread it on your wet skin, concentrating on any calluses on your feet, elbows, or knees. Use the cream to smooth and polish your shoulders, arms, thighs, hips, and torso. Rub the buffing cream gently in a rotating motion, using your hands or a washcloth. Avoid irritated areas, skin that has broken out, and very thin or fragile skin — the underarms, breasts, groin, and inner thighs. Then, using light massaging movements with your hands or washcloth, rinse away all traces of buffing cream. If you have especially stubborn calluses or hard skin on your feet, elbows, hands, or knees, use the cream regularly on these particular areas.

Buffing is the second important step in your total body skin-care routine. Faithful use of a buffing cream will help your skin function healthfully and look and feel extra clean, soft, and lustrous.

Like polishing your skin, buffing with a cream shines your shoulders, gives legs and hips a silken luster, and softens calluses on heels and elbows. And as it invigorates, it sloughs off dull surface cells. Buffed skin looks clearer, softer, and smoother and makes you feel wonderful about the special care you're giving your body.

oisturize

A square inch of your body skin has fewer oil glands than an area of facial skin the same size, so it may dry out easily no matter what your skin type. Body skin is also subject to much abuse. Tight or binding clothing can rub and irritate your skin. Shaving legs and underarms (see pages 202 and 203), because it allows moisture to evaporate from the skin, can contribute to dryness. To substitute for lost natural oils on your body skin, you should regularly apply a rich, creamy moisturizing lotion that disappears completely. A moisturizer should make your skin smooth and supple, with no greasy after-feel, and leave a fresh scent that won't interfere with other fragrances.

How and When to Moisturize After your shower or bath, gently towel dry your body, leaving it slightly damp. Pour a generous amount of body moisturizer into your hand and smooth it all over. When applied to damp skin, body moisturizer helps hold some water on the skin's surface. Massage the lotion gently onto your skin, covering your shoulders, chest, arms, waist, stomach, hips, buttocks, and legs. Pay special attention to drier areas, such as your lower arms, lower legs, feet, elbows, and knees. Continue spreading the lotion evenly all over until it disappears completely.

Moisturize as often as you feel your body skin requires it; at least several times a week is recommended. Use body moisturizing lotion after every bath or shower on drier areas of your body, or in winter, when skin tends to be drier. Use the lotion as often and as liberally as you like, especially on dry areas. If your skin is unusually sensitive, however, avoid irritated or just-shaved areas.

A body moisturizing lotion that helps protect your skin from moisture loss is the important third step in your consistent program of total body care.

Your skin needs moisture to function well and look its best, and a body moisturizing lotion helps your skin retain its precious beautifying moisture. Smooth moisturizer over arms, legs, shoulders, torso — everywhere — after your shower or bath for soft, velvety skin.

Protect

Heat, cold, environmental dryness, and, in particular, damaging effects of the sun can all contribute to aging skin. To counteract the potential dangers of the environment, you should regularly use a sunscreening lotion with moisturizing agents.

If you engage in active sports or swimming, your sunscreening lotion should be water-resistant and have a sun protection factor (SPF) of at least 10. Whatever your skin type, you need a sunscreen that helps shield your body from the sun's harmful ultraviolet rays and slows down premature aging caused by overexposure. This protective lotion should leave no greasy after-feel.

How and When to Protect Use your sunscreening lotion whenever you are going to be out in the sun. Apply it evenly to clean skin on all uncovered areas of your body. Sunscreen is most effective when you apply it seven to fifteen minutes before going outdoors. Reapply after swimming or strenuous exercise, or if you perspire heavily. Sunscreening lotion may be applied over body moisturizing lotion.

Slow tanning will still occur through a sunscreen. Your body sunscreening lotion functions to help protect your skin from harmful ultraviolet radiation. Even with a sunscreen, however, it's best not to "bake" in the sun for long periods of time, especially between the hours of 10 A.M. and 2 P.M. (11 A.M. to 3 P.M. daylight saving time) when the sun's rays are strongest.

Protecting your skin is the fourth essential step in your all-over, total body skin care. Remember: damage from sun exposure is permanent and irreversible, so it is essential that you include this step in your body skin-care routine.

Protecting your skin from the sun's damaging rays is the fourth step in your body-care routine. Smooth sunscreen over uncovered skin when you're outdoors, for a softer, younger-looking body.

$\mathscr{Y}$ear-Round Sun Protection

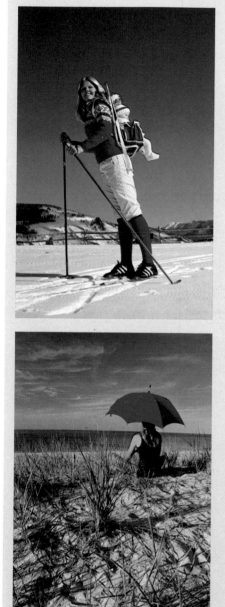

Because your skin is exposed to ultraviolet radiation from the sun whenever you are outdoors, a body sunscreening lotion is important throughout the year, not just on summer days at the beach.

The more distant **winter** sun can be misleading. It's especially important to protect all exposed body skin whenever there is snow — while skiing, ice skating, sledding, or walking, particularly in the mountains where high altitudes intensify the effects of ultraviolet radiation. Snow reflects up to 85 percent of the sun's rays, making the dangers of sun damage even greater in snow conditions than at the beach. In winter, urban areas are also potentially dangerous, as many glass- or mirror-covered buildings reflect sunlight. Use a sunscreening lotion whenever you plan to be outdoors for long periods of time, even in the absence of bright sunshine. Your skin will be exposed to damaging ultraviolet radiation even if the sun isn't shining.

Autumn is a season we are often outdoors, but because the air seems cool, we may not notice prolonged exposure to sunlight. Remember: damaging ultraviolet rays don't feel warm. Use a sunscreening lotion on all exposed body skin whenever you plan to be outside in the fall.

Protection is most critical during the **summer** because the sun is strongest and outdoor activities most popular. Use sunscreening lotion whenever you will be outside: playing sports such as tennis or golf; attending social events such as picnics or barbecues; even gardening or walking to work. If you perspire heavily, reapply your sunscreen often. Even when the sky is hazy, ultraviolet radiation is still strong, increasing the danger of overexposure because you may not be aware of the intensity of the sun's rays. Those who live in high altitudes should take even greater precaution. At the beach, use sunscreening lotion on hazy or sunny days. Sand reflects as much as 17 percent of the sun's rays and intensifies exposure.

Skin damage from sun exposure can occur in the **spring** when the air is still apt to be cool and you do not feel heat rays right away. Protect all exposed body skin with your body sunscreening lotion whenever you plan to be outdoors.

Hand Care

Beautiful hands result from proper, ongoing care. They reflect your commitment to grooming, an unmistakable sign that you pay attention to the details of your appearance. The first step in nail care is correcting minor flaws. Here are some solutions:

Nails that chip, break, peel, or split can be mended with a variety of products available for home use. Nail hardeners, which can be used as a base or top coat, help harden and protect weak, soft nails. However, these must be used with great caution because of their strong chemicals. Discontinue use if you suspect an allergic reaction. Nail wrapping strengthens nails and extends the life of nail polish. Both nail hardeners and nail wrapping give long nails extra protection. To prevent nails from *tearing at the sides,* file only the nail edge to round off the tips.

Ridges can be treated with a special ridge-filling product and a nail-smoothing board. These items even out the ridges as the nail grows out and help prepare the nail surface for polish. (Prominent or new ridges can be symptomatic of an underlying medical problem; consult a doctor.) *White spots,* air spaces in the nail or tiny bruises under the surface, also grow out with the nail. To hide white spots, coat them with opaque nail enamel.

Ragged, uneven cuticles can be prevented by making cuticle care part of your nightly routine. Massage in cuticle conditioner to guard against cracking and drying. Soak your nails weekly in warm, sudsy water, then follow with cuticle conditioner. Next, push back cuticles gently with the rounded end of a manicure stick. Don't trim your cuticles with nail scissors or cuticle nippers; recent evidence indicates that trimming destroys the protective function of the cuticle and can lead to inflammation and infections in the nail bed.

Nail stains can be removed by buffing, which also increases blood circulation. A base coat applied prior to polish helps prevent the enamel color from staining the nail.

You can prevent polish from *bubbling* if you apply it carefully. Make sure your nails are clean, dry, and free of oil, and allow each coat of polish to dry thoroughly. Brush on polish away from direct heat or air-conditioning vents. If polish gets too thick, thin it with a nail enamel thinner. Finally, give freshly polished nails a chance to dry completely. If you don't have time to let them dry naturally, be sure to use a liquid or aerosol drying product.

Tips for Pretty Hands

To protect hands in cold, dry weather, use a rich hand cream with added sunscreen, and always wear gloves outdoors. Carry a purse-sized container of lotion with you and moisturize your hands several times a day.

Since hot water, household cleansing products, and detergents can be extremely drying, wear rubber gloves when you do housework, especially washing dishes. (Keep a pair by the sink to remind you.) For extra moisturization, apply hand cream before putting on gloves.

Heavy work — such as gardening or outdoor chores — calls for heavy gloves to protect skin and nails. Also, if you play golf or racquet sports, try to prevent calluses by wearing the special gloves designed for these purposes.

Always carry an emery board in your purse in case a nail breaks or tears. Rough edges look unsightly and can catch on your clothing.

Everything you need to take care of your hands is, so to speak, right at your fingertips. Your lifestyle and personal preference affect the length you keep your nails and the shade of polish you choose. However, once you achieve the look you want, maintenance takes just a small amount of time each week. Here's how to give yourself a manicure.

Manicure Tools
Nail polish remover and cotton balls
Emery board
Shallow bowl for soaking your fingertips
Cleansing gel
Clean, soft hand towel
Manicure stick
Cuticle conditioner
Ridge filler and nail buffer (optional)
Base coat, nail polish, top coat
Hand cream

1 Remove old polish with nail polish remover and cotton balls, then file and shape your nails. Use a file instead of nail scissors because cutting can weaken your nails. With an emery board, file your nails in one direction, toward the center. Don't saw the emery board back and forth across the edges of your nails, as this can roughen the surface.

2 Put warm water and cleansing gel into a shallow bowl and soak your fingers for about a minute. As you dry your hands, gently loosen any dirt with a manicure stick.

3 Apply cuticle conditioner along your cuticles. Push back cuticles gently with the blunt, rounded end of a manicure stick. (These sticks are ideal for cuticles and under nails because they are made of soft wood that won't tear or damage the fragile cuticle and under-nail skin.)

4 Depending on your needs, apply ridge filler and/or buff your nails. Always buff nails at an angle in one direction. If you wish to apply polish, remove all traces of cuticle conditioner by patting nails dry with a towel. Nails should be free of oil before you apply polish. Brush on a base coat and allow it to dry. Then apply nail enamel with three quick strokes from the base to the tip — one down the middle of the nail and one on each side. Apply two or three times, allowing each coat to dry between applications. Finish with a top coat; for extra protection, brush it under the tips of your nails. Again, allow it to dry. (You may want to use a special nail-drying product at this time.) To keep hands feeling soft and smooth, rub in hand cream. For extra protection, choose one with added sunscreen.

Foot Care

You may not think of including your feet in your regular beauty routine. After all, they're not as visible as the rest of your body. But proper foot care offers many benefits: it completes your head-to-toe beauty look and enhances the appearance of your feet in bare, strappy sandals. It also helps guard against minor foot problems that can leave feet sore or unsightly. Perhaps most important of all, well-cared-for feet make you feel good.

To keep your feet in peak condition, buff and moisturize them regularly. This is especially useful on heels and soles, where calluses are likely to develop. For feet that look and feel sensational, give yourself a pedicure — once a month in cool weather and once every two weeks in warm weather.

Pedicure Tools

Nail polish remover and cotton balls	Soft nailbrush
Toenail clipper	Clean, soft towel
Emery board	Moisturizer
Large basin or bowl	Cuticle conditioner
Cleansing gel	Manicure stick
Pumice stone	Tissue or foam rubber separators
	Base coat, nail polish, top coat

Remove old polish with nail polish remover and cotton balls. Trim your toenails with a toenail clipper; refer to the box at left for the proper procedure. Then use an emery board to smooth rough edges and corners.

Put warm water and cleansing gel in a large basin and soak your feet for ten minutes. Use a pumice stone dipped in the water to soften rough skin and calluses. (Regular use of buffing cream in the bath or shower also helps smooth and soften feet.)

With a soft nailbrush dipped in the water, scrub your toenails lightly to loosen dirt and buff your nails. Towel your feet dry.

Apply cuticle conditioner along your cuticles. Push them back gently with the rounded end of a manicure stick. Clean under nails with the pointed end.

If you wish to apply nail polish, separate your toes with tissue or a foam-rubber separator. Begin with a base coat, then follow with two or three coats of polish. (A manicure stick is handy for cleaning smears of polish on the skin around your nails.) Be sure to allow ample drying time between applications. Apply the top coat and allow your nails to dry completely before removing the separators.

Finish by massaging in moisturizer. Begin with your toes, then spread moisturizer over your feet, on your legs, and down again. Rub it well into the soles of your feet.

Trimming Toenails

Using a nail clipper, cut each toenail *straight across,* following the shape of your toe. Toenails should be even with — never longer than — the ends of your toes. But don't cut them too short because the tender flesh under your nails is not meant to be exposed.

Smooth jagged edges with the dark, coarse side of an emery board. Then use the light, fine side to finish smoothing your cut nail edges. Be sure to move the emery board in one direction, toward the center.

Tips for Pretty Feet

Buy shoes carefully. Check the length and width, and be sure shoes fit well at the heel. Toes should have room to move freely, and uppers should not cause friction when you walk. To get the most accurate fit, shop for shoes at the end of the day when your feet are most swollen. Finally, avoid buying shoes that need "breaking in" — you'll most likely have problems with them later on.

Vary heel heights regularly to help tone calf muscles while soothing heels and soles.

Elevate your feet for a few minutes each day to improve circulation.

Refresh tired feet with a lightly scented talc.

Avoid walking barefoot on hard surfaces; it hardens skin and promotes calluses. However, walking barefoot on sand can be beneficial — sand acts as a natural pumice for your feet.

air Removal

Hair grows all over the body in varying amounts, distribution, and texture. Your quota of body hair is principally a factor of heredity, but excess growth may in some cases be related to hormonal imbalance or medication. If, as an adult, you notice sudden body hair growth in any area, it's best to consult a physician regarding the cause. Many women are concerned about unwanted hair growth on their legs, under their arms, and on other parts of their bodies. The methods for removing this hair range from professional treatments for permanent removal to home treatments that take it off temporarily or make it less noticeable. Hair removal should be a part of your personal grooming routine; how you accomplish it depends on the area of the body you are dealing with and on your individual needs and preferences.

Electrolysis can be a safe and effective method of permanently removing hair from the body. This technique destroys the hair root through an electric current. A very fine wire needle is inserted into the opening of the hair follicle, and an electric current is transmitted down the needle to destroy the root. Each hair then falls out or is removed with tweezers. Since each hair is individually treated, it takes a long time to remove a lot of hair by this process. Electrolysis may also be costly and uncomfortable, so you should consider it only for removing hair in small areas — your upper lip or chin, between your breasts, or surrounding your navel. Because of possible scarring (if excess current is used) and infection (if equipment is not sterile), it is extremely important to choose a competent professional electrologist. Ask your dermatologist for a recommendation.

Tweezing is a semipermanent method of hair removal. It removes the hair by pulling out the root, and it takes a long time for the hair to grow back. Because it is slightly uncomfortable and tedious, tweezing is not recommended for large areas of body hair, but it may be suitable for stray hairs between your breasts or near your navel, as well as for minor facial hair problems. (Never tweeze hair from a mole or mark on your skin — consult a dermatologist.)

Depilatories — over-the-counter chemical compounds — dissolve or loosen surface hair. You apply a depilatory to your skin, leaving it on for a specified amount of time. When you wipe off the cream, the hair should come off with it. But chemicals strong

Hair growth on legs and underarms comes off easily with the whisk of a razor when you use body cleansing gel to soften your skin and reduce surface friction. Shaving is one of several grooming options for removing unwanted hair.

enough to break down the composition of body hair may also irritate your skin. Before you use a home depilatory product, test it on a small, less sensitive area of your body — the tougher skin on your arms or legs. Milder depilatories, specially formulated for hair on the facial skin, are best for this sensitive area. Regrowth after use of a depilatory may take from two to three weeks, although some hairs grow in faster than others.

Waxing is another technique for hair removal that lasts about two to three weeks; it may be less irritating to your skin than chemical depilatories. Warm wax is spread on the area from which hair is to be removed, allowed to dry, then pulled off in hard strips to which the hair adheres. Waxing is suitable for many areas of the body, including the face, and is especially effective for arm, leg, and even underarm hair.

Shaving is the least permanent method of hair removal, since hair may reappear within twenty-four hours. But shaving is an extremely effective and easy method for temporarily removing hair from your lower legs and underarms. A foaming, moisturizing product like body cleansing gel helps a razor glide easily over your skin to remove hair in the bath or shower and helps prevent the dryness that often accompanies shaving. Use of body moisturizing lotion on your lower legs after shaving also helps keep them silky smooth and well conditioned. Your upper thighs and bikini line may not respond well to shaving; regrowth may cause irritation and ingrown hairs.

Bleaching with creams or lotions lightens the color of body hair by chemically lifting the pigment so that the paler color of the hair blends with the skin and is less noticeable. Since bleaching alters the structure of the hair by penetrating the cuticle and tends to make hair coarser, it is best used on only the finest, sparsest growth; also, patch tests are recommended on areas where the product is to be applied to determine whether it will cause irritation. Hair on your arms, legs, and, if needed, bikini line may be bleached effectively. Regrowth of darker roots generally occurs within a week.

regnancy and You

Hormonal changes that accompany pregnancy affect the way your skin looks and feels, not only on your face but elsewhere on your body. Your skin may become oilier; frequent cleansing with a mild cleansing gel helps. Skin that becomes dry during pregnancy may look and feel less dehydrated through frequent use of body moisture lotion after a bath or shower. Exposure to the sun may cause irregular spotting of body skin during pregnancy, so it is especially important to protect your skin with a sunscreening lotion whenever you are going to be outdoors.

Cholestasis of pregnancy is an itchy condition that results when an increased hormonal level affects the liver. Changes in circulation during pregnancy may cause fine-lined, weblike veins to show through the surface of the skin on your arms, hands, neck, upper chest, or face. These tend to disappear shortly after delivery.

Your body skin may also be affected by physical changes that occur during pregnancy. Because enlargement of the uterus puts pressure on the large blood vessels in the pelvis, veins in the legs sometimes become dilated, and the extremities swell. In some cases, varicose veins develop and persist after pregnancy. To prevent this condition, it is usually recommended that pregnant women keep their legs elevated as much as possible. (If you develop varicose veins, cosmetic surgical treatments are available to remove them.)

Stretch marks are possibly the most prevalent and bothersome of all body skin conditions related to pregnancy. The American Academy of Dermatology estimates that as many as 90 percent of all women develop these marks, which are caused by the pulling and separating of collagen and elastin tissues below the skin's surface, usually on the thighs, buttocks, breasts, and abdomen. Topical creams or oils cannot prevent or help these marks, since the problem originates in the lower layer of the skin. Certain measures may help avoid the development of stretch marks, however; a pregnancy panty girdle helps provide support for the tissues of the abdomen and buttocks, for example, and mild exercises can increase muscle tone in the affected areas. If you develop stretch marks despite your precautions, you may be able to conceal them with body makeup.

Throughout your pregnancy, your personal physician is your best source for all related information. He or she can offer all the advice

Your pregnancy is a beautiful time in your life — especially when you maximize all the beautifying health benefits of good body care. Now more than ever you'll want to do everything you can for your overall health.

you need regarding your skin's condition, the amount of exercise you need, and the best diet for you. Although an active pregnancy is now considered healthy for many women, it may not be suitable for you individually. Consult your doctor before you begin any type of exercise program or regular sports activity while you're pregnant.

In many cases, pregnancy enhances a woman's beauty, giving her an all-over glow that is characteristic of this very special time in her life. It can be an excellent time to make the most of the way you look and feel, a prime opportunity to take care of yourself and be your healthy best.

Nutrition and You

How important is proper nutrition to looking and feeling your best? The answer becomes increasingly clear when you consider the key role a balanced and healthy diet plays in:

- your appearance — your skin, hair, nails, teeth, muscle strength, weight, even under-eye circles
- your energy level
- your moods
- your overall health and well-being

The following tips will help you get maximum benefit from the foods you eat.

1. Eat a variety of foods. For optimum nutrition, you need a balanced diet that includes foods from all four major food groups: milk and dairy products; meat, fish, poultry, and eggs; fruits and vegetables; and breads and cereals. Note that certain choices within these groups provide especially high nutritional value: low-fat milk, low-fat cheese, and low-fat yogurt; salmon, haddock, halibut, chicken (skin removed), kidney beans, and eggs; apples, bananas, broccoli, carrots, spinach, and strawberries; and whole-grain bread, brown rice, and bran muffins.

2. Get the most nutritional value from your food. The way you choose and prepare foods is important to getting the best nutritional value. Good habits to adopt include:
   - reading labels to determine which foods offer the most nutrients for the calories
   - planning meals in advance to avoid impulse eating
   - preparing foods in the most nutritious manner, such as baking instead of frying, trimming off excess fat, and steaming vegetables instead of boiling

3. Keep carbohydrates, proteins, and fats in balance. All three are important; the key is keeping the ratio you consume in balance — approximately 55 to 65 percent carbohydrates, 10 to 15 percent protein, and 25 to 35 percent fat.

4. Include fiber in your diet. Fiber, an indigestible carbohydrate, is important for controlling and regulating the process of food ab-

Apples, a healthy alternative to snacks containing refined sugar, provide longer-lasting energy as well as fiber.

sorption and is believed to help guard against certain types of cancer and coronary disease. Among those foods highest in fiber you'll want to include in your diet are whole-wheat bread, high-fiber cereals, kidney beans, brown rice, peas, blackberries, pears, and apples.

5. Get the recommended amount of calcium. Medical experts have cited a relationship between women's low calcium intake and osteoporosis, a condition of too little bone mass which can cause bones to become weak and brittle. Among those high-calcium foods you'll want to include in your diet are low-fat dairy products, sardines, salmon, sunflower seeds, soybeans, and leafy green vegetables.

Vitamins and You

The question of whether you can benefit from taking vitamin and mineral supplements is determined by a range of factors. First, you need to look at such basic and relatively stable factors as your inherited biochemistry, age, sex, metabolic rate, and body weight. Equally important are more variable factors, which can be divided into three main categories — nutritional habits, amount of physical activity, and lifestyle. The following list will help you identify some of the habits and activities that may prevent you from getting the proper amounts of certain vitamins and minerals — and, as a result, increase your need for vitamin supplementation.

- skipping meals
- eating out frequently (particularly fast food)
- dieting (including vegetarian diets)
- regular exercise
- caffeine and alcohol consumption
- smoking
- medication and/or use of oral contraceptives
- stress

Why do you need vitamins and minerals? Vitamins and minerals are essential to nerve, muscle, and brain function as well as a vital part of the metabolic chain — the process whereby food is broken down and used as energy. In order for these biochemical processes to run at peak efficiency, you need both the proper variety and amounts of nutrients. Because food alone often fails to provide adequate supplies of vitamins and minerals, vitamin supplements can act as insurance, helping to compensate for dietary shortages.

What is the required amount of vitamins and minerals? The Recommended Dietary Allowances (RDAs) of vitamins and minerals, prepared by the Food and Nutrition Board of the National Academy of Sciences, is a government estimate of the amounts healthy people should eat daily. The accompanying chart, developed in 1980, provides the RDA, function, and natural food sources of selected vitamins and minerals.

Vitamin and Mineral Requirements and Function

Vitamins	Recommended Daily Dietary Allowance	Function	Food Sources
A	5,000 IU*	Bone growth, teeth development, healthy skin and hair	Leafy green and yellow vegetables, liver, eggs, milk
D	400 IU	Helps form and maintain bones and teeth	Milk, eggs, tuna, salmon
E	30 IU	Helps form red blood cells, muscles, and other tissues	Grains, wheat germ, sunflower and vegetable oils
K	.07–.14 mg*	Blood clotting	Lentils, yogurt, molasses, leafy green vegetables
B-1	1.5 mg	Helps release energy from carbohydrates	Cereals, lean meats, poultry, fish, liver, pork
B-2	1.7 mg	Helps release energy from carbohydrates, proteins, and fats; respiration	Cereals, lean meats, yeast, eggs, leafy green vegetables
B-3 (Niacin)	13–18 mg	Helps generate energy for normal cell function	Chicken, pork, fish, yeast, roasted peanuts
B-6	2 mg	Aids absorption and metabolism of proteins; helps body use fat; helps form red blood cells	Cereals, bananas, yeast, meat, wheat germ, vegetables
B-12	3 mg	Helps form red blood cells, maintains nervous system, build genetic material	Fish, lean meat, liver, milk
C	60 mg	Helps form collagen; maintains capillaries, bones, and teeth; accelerates healing	Citrus fruits, leafy green vegetables, berries, tomatoes, cauliflower, cabbage

Minerals

Minerals	Recommended Daily Dietary Allowance	Function	Food Sources
Calcium	800–1,000 mg	Bone formation and structure; helps maintain teeth	Milk, cheese, nuts, green vegetables
Iron	10–18 mg	Healthy blood; helps prevent fatigue	Whole-grain cereals, nuts, green vegetables, oysters, liver
Phosphorous	800–1,200 mg	Bone formation and structure; helps body use fats, proteins, and carbohydrates	Eggs, fish, meat, poultry, grains, cheese
Magnesium	300–400 mg	Bone formation and structure; muscle relaxation	Whole grains, seafood, green vegetables, nuts, lemons, grapefruit
Zinc	15 mg	Cell division, repair, and growth; bone growth and development	Yeast, whole grains, liver, sunflower seeds
Iodine	150 mcg*	Thyroid production and metabolism	Seafood, kelp, iodized salt

*IU stands for international unit; mg stands for milligram; mcg stands for microgram (one-thousandth of a milligram).

xercise and You

An essential part of total beauty is an overall feeling of well-being — the ability to relax, set priorities, and manage any setbacks. You want to balance the many aspects of your life, to fulfill your responsibilities yet still have time to devote to yourself. Most important, you need to make a commitment to feeling good — physically and psychologically. Specifically, this means developing positive, healthy habits: getting enough sleep, exercising regularly, eating properly. It also means setting goals that are challenging yet realistic.

Exercise   There are so many reasons to keep your body in top condition. The most obvious is you'll look sensational. Most likely you'll also feel more energized, be more alert, raise your self-confidence, and be able to handle stress more effectively. And as an extra bonus, you may help reduce your susceptibility to certain diseases. Quite simply, exercise is one activity that guarantees you a return on your investment.

There's an exercise to suit just about every interest, lifestyle, and skill level. Naturally, you'll want to choose something you enjoy, whether it's jogging, swimming, ballet, aerobic dancing, or any of countless other activities. The key is to focus on what you can do, not on what you can't.

Start at a comfortable level and build up gradually; never overdo exercise at the beginning. Keep in mind, however, that for any exercise program to be effective, you must stick with it — vigorously and consistently. When you begin to see results, you'll be encouraged to progress even further.

In addition, you want to make a conscious effort to build movement into your day-to-day activities. Climb stairs. Walk to work, or from the train station or bus stop. Ride your bike to do errands. Bend and stretch when you do everyday household chores. (Be sure to bend your knees when lifting heavy objects to avoid straining your back.) Whenever possible, be a participant rather than a spectator. Once you begin, you'll be amazed at all the opportunities to add exercise to your schedule.

As you set up your individual program, try to combine a number of different exercises and activities. This will work the greatest number of muscle groups and, at the same time, give your routine variety. Aim to include at least twenty minutes of vigorous, sustained

Exercise keeps you trim, fit, and toned — and it makes you feel wonderfully alive. Jumping rope is an excellent aerobic activity that increases circulation and oxygen exchange. This form of exercise can improve your overall strength and stamina and help tone your muscles.

aerobic exercise (activities that increase your oxygen intake and heart rate) at least three times a week: among the possibilities are aerobic dance class, jogging, bicycling, swimming, jumping rope, and cross-country skiing.

To supplement your aerobic workout, you can add sports, spot exercises, and overall stretching to your routine. You'll help firm and tone as you increase your flexibility and coordination. In addition, you might consider joining a health club in your area. Many offer excellent programs for all-around fitness along with such extras as whirlpools, saunas, racquetball and tennis courts, exercise classes, and child-care facilities. No matter what, always check with your doctor before beginning any kind of exercise program.

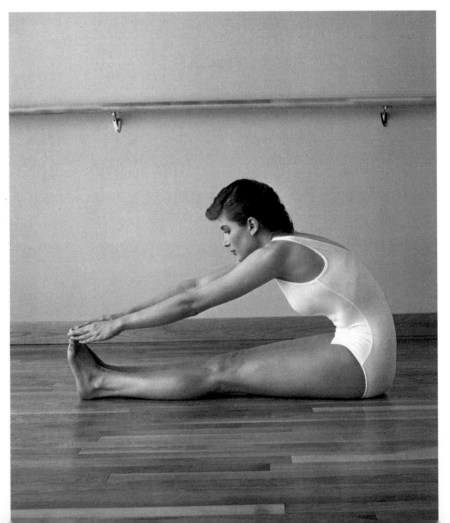

A fit, firm body is worth working for. Weight lifting tones and firms your muscles and improves your coordination and motor skills. Stretching is a mild form of exercise that tones and extends your muscles, strengthens your spine, and increases your flexibility. It can help relieve tension and is excellent for warming up before aerobic exercise or sports.

Sleep, Relaxation, and You

Sleep You spend about one-third of your life sleeping — so naturally you want to make those hours count. A good night's sleep offers a number of beauty benefits: it can help you feel more alert and alive, it can increase your energy level, and it can make it seem as though you're able to fit more into your day.

How much sleep do you need? Six to eight hours is considered the norm for healthy adults, although your individual needs may vary. And along with the quantity, the quality of your sleep is important. Choose a mattress that gives you the support you need (many experts recommend a mattress that's on the firm side, although you may want to check with your doctor). To elevate the neck properly, one pillow is generally suggested.

Another key consideration is the climate you sleep in. Personal comfort is the first guideline, although some sleep studies indicate the best temperature for sleep is between 64 and 68 degrees Fahrenheit. Avoid rooms that are too dry; mucous membranes can dry out and make breathing more difficult. If dryness is a problem, a humidifier may help, especially in winter.

You'll sleep better, too, if you avoid heavy eating and exercise before bed. Other relaxers include light reading, yoga, and progressive relaxation. And don't overlook the importance of your surroundings. Make your bedroom a comfortable, enjoyable place to be. The best environment for sleep is a room that reflects your personal and very special needs and tastes.

Relaxation No matter how much you fit into your daily schedule, it's essential to work in time for relaxation. Setting aside a few minutes to break from your routine can increase productivity and lift the spirits; it can also help you manage stress.

There is, however, no one relaxation technique that will work for everyone. Some women, for example, may find a leisurely bath, a long walk, or a brisk jog relaxing; others may get the desired results with yoga, meditation, massage, or progressive relaxation. The key is to experiment with different methods — to discover what will refresh *your* mind and relieve *your* tension. Once you find the right activity — or combination of activities — you'll discover the positive effects relaxation can have on your life.

It's important for everyone to take time to preserve interests that are special and provide time alone.

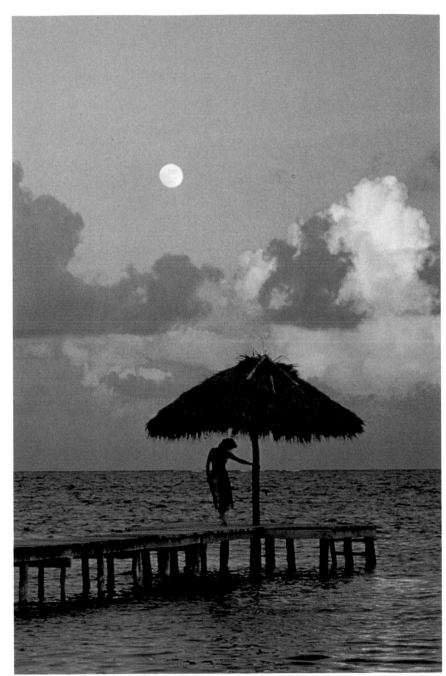

Whether it's an hour's walk on the beach, a hike in the woods, or some pensive time alone in a favorite spot, it's good to get outdoors on a regular basis.

ragrance

It is estimated that the use of fragrance goes back at least six thousand years. Priests first used perfumes as offerings to the gods; in time, they used them as healing oils. Fragrance later evolved into an element of personal grooming as the nobility of both sexes applied scented oils to increase their attractiveness and allure. But fragrance has never been as popular as it is today.

Formulas for fragrances have been developed over the ages, from simple perfumed oils, to oils blended with alcohol, to today's complex scents. Think of the vast array of aromatic materials that go into a single fragrance: fresh flowers that create soft floral notes; bright citrus scents derived from lemon, orange, and lime; tree moss used to create sensuous mossy tones; spicy notes derived from blending cinnamon, clove, nutmeg, and pepper; rosemary, sage, and basil, which add fresh herbaceous scents; woodsy aromas from sandalwood, cedar, and rosewood; myrrh and fir, which add heady, incenselike scents; even man-made ingredients that simulate natural aromatics. How are these various aromas combined to create the sophisticated perfumes that women use today?

The creation of fragrance is both art and science. Those who blend fragrances are trained scientists with very special talents. The person who assembles a final formula for fragrance is called a master perfumer, or "nose." He or she is trained to distinguish the various combinations of materials that go into fragrances — a skill that takes years of study. During this time the master perfumer also develops an acute and sophisticated sense of smell.

The creator of a fragrance selects ingredients for a fragrance from over five thousand natural and/or aromatic materials. These materials, which come from all over the world, can be extremely expensive. For example, jasmine, which blooms only at night, must be picked within a few hours of blooming, while the petals are still open. Roses must be gathered at sunrise, when they are still moist with dew; four thousand pounds of rose petals are required to make a single pound of the rose oil that goes into a variety of fragrances. Flowers used for floral fragrances must be picked by hand, and it takes one person an entire eight-hour day to pick about fifty pounds of flowers.

Since the eighteenth century, the town of Grasse, in southern France, has been a primary source of flowers for perfume. The warm climate in this area is ideal for growing and harvesting natural jasmine, rose, tuberose, and other flowers used for floral notes in fragrances. During the nineteenth century, when Paris became the fashion capital of the world, prestigious perfume houses were established, and France became famous for its production of fine fragrances. Since then, other countries, including the United States, have found their own distinctive blends of scents to create unique fragrances. Today, fragrances may be made wherever in the world there are materials to create them.

The creation of a fragrance requires a long and careful process of combining many different materials. A fragrance you respond to in a matter of minutes often has taken years to create.

Although fragrance by its nature is ephemeral, it can leave a lasting impression of its wearer. In any single fragrance scores of ingredients combine to create a scent that, when it reacts with your body's chemistry, will become your personal signature.

Fragrance

Buying a fragrance is different from buying any other personal item. Purchasing fragrance is an emotional experience, for perfumes can express moods and evoke special feelings and memories. You cannot evaluate fragrances by smelling them in the bottle or admiring their aroma on someone else. You must choose your favorites by trying them on and allowing them to blend with the unique chemistry of your skin oils and moisture.

To test a fragrance, apply a few drops to your inner wrist. Allow them to dry, then pass your wrist back and forth several inches from your nose. The first impression you receive, the most identifiable of the combined scents, is called the *top note*. A fragrance's top note is its brightest — fresh, fervent, and volatile.

Sniff your wrist after ten minutes, holding it close to — but not touching — your nose. As a fragrance begins to blend with your body chemistry, the essence reaches its deepest intensity. The second impression you receive is of the *middle note,* the mellow heart of the fragrance. At this point you can decide whether you like the impression of the fragrance.

You may not notice the lingering *bottom note* of a fragrance until two to three hours after you apply it. Bring your inner wrist up to your nose and inhale deeply. This — the final impression, generally composed of wood, moss, or musk scents — is of the aroma those around you will smell. In some fragrances these three stages may not be noticeable, but in others they will be obvious.

Sample fragrances in midmorning, when your sense of smell is most accurate, and at least several hours after eating, for spicy foods can alter your sense of smell. Since it is difficult to evaluate a great variety of scents at the same time, limit your selection to two possibilities, sampling one fragrance on each wrist.

Your selection of a fragrance should be based on your evaluation of how it suits your personality, your moods, and your preferences. The most important factor in buying fragrance, however, is how well you like the way a particular scent reacts with your unique body chemistry. The same fragrance never smells the same on any two women, so you can choose a fragrance and make it yours. And don't limit yourself to a single selection. Build a wardrobe of fragrances for all the moods and occasions in your life.

Fragrances not only smell wonderful, they come in elegant, beautiful bottles. Display yours in a convenient location so they're always within reach.

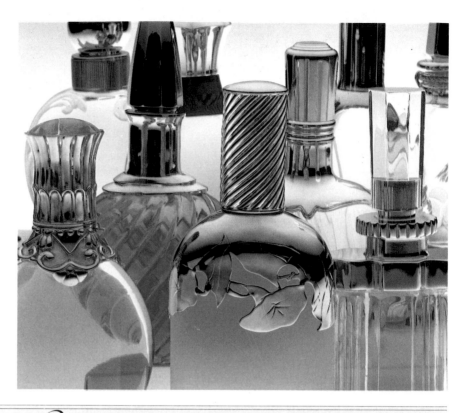

ℳaking Sense of Scents

Once you've chosen your favorites, how much of these fragrances you should wear depends on the kind of impact you want to make, the mood you wish to impart, the ambience of scent you want to surround you. Subtle and fleeting? Direct and dramatic? Mysteriously atmospheric? Your choice may depend on the time of day, your mood of the moment, the occasion, or the people you'll meet.

Fragrance strength may depend on the *type* of scent you select (Oriental scents are the most powerful and longest lasting), but it also depends directly on the form of fragrance you use.

Of all the liquid forms of scent, *perfume* has the highest concentration of fragrance oil in ratio to the alcohol with which it is blended. The most expensive form of fragrance, perfume is the strongest and dressiest, and it lingers longest. A touch of perfume at pulse points will surround you with scent when you want to feel ultrafeminine.

Eau de toilette in the French tradition ranks second in strength, as more alcohol and sometimes water are used to dilute the fragrance oils; with its greater proportion of alcohol, eau de toilette evaporates more quickly over time. You may want to use more of it over your body skin for immediate fragrance impact, but you'll need to reapply eau de toilette throughout the day or evening to keep your scent fresh and strong. Eau de toilette is a versatile form of fragrance that's just right when you want a long-lasting fragrance for an active lifestyle.

Cologne in the French tradition — which has the lowest ratio of fragrance oils to alcohol and water — is the most fleeting liquid form of scent. Cologne may be splashed or sprayed on lavishly, but you'll need to repeat applications often if you want continuous, all-day fragrance. With its minimal lingering power, cologne is appropriate for your moods, occasions, and roles that call for light scents. Just the right touch for your business or daytime image, cologne can be reapplied for extra impact after five.

Scented bath products — soaps, powders, talcs, lotions, and milk baths — provide just a hint of soft fragrance. They are intended for your quietest, most subtle fragrance needs or as basic underlayers for more intense forms of fragrance.

Fragrance

There are as many reasons to wear fragrance as there are ways to wear it. A fresh, lighthearted fragrance can lift your spirits just when they need it. A spray of the right scent can make you feel romantic, feminine, and sensuous. Fragrance can evoke mystery or add drama. It can make you feel luxurious and elegant or winsome and lively. Fragrance creates an impression that becomes part of your total beauty. You can wear one fragrance so only a single scent is clearly identified with you. Or you can experiment with a variety of fragrances to suit your mood or the occasion.

Choose your fragrance with the same careful thought you apply to your wardrobe. Use a fresh, bright, sporty fragrance for days when you're dressed casually, then switch to a dramatically intense scent when you dress up in the evening.

Layer your fragrances to increase their holding power and create different impressions of scent as the day or evening wears on. Start with a rich cream bath fragrance in your bathwater, then puff on matching talc or dusting powder. Spray the same fragrance of cologne under the hair at the back of your neck, on your shoulders, and at your waist. Then dab on matching perfume at pulse points: your inner wrists, behind your ears, behind your knees, at the base of your neck, and inside your elbows. Carry a purse-sized spray cologne or perfume with you for touch-ups during the day or evening.

Use your fragrances creatively. Make a sachet by saturating a cotton ball with your favorite fragrance and place it in a closet or dresser drawer. Fragrance can also be sprayed on dried flower arrangements or in lined dresser drawers to add a whisper of scent to linens. Place empty bottles in lingerie drawers to add a delicate scent to your underclothes.

Fragrance is the ideal way to be good to yourself, to make yourself feel special — and let others know you're special. Wear it to enhance your mood, to express who you are, what you like, how you feel. Make fragrance a part of your personal beauty statement every day — the finishing touch to a perfectly groomed and totally beautiful you.

Apply fragrance at the base of your throat, on your wrists, behind your knees, or on any of your pulse points — where your skin's chemistry combines beautifully with your scent to surround you with sensual aromas.

Jennifer is a homemaker and mother with two small children to care for. Her days are full of responsibilities; they start early and are busy throughout. Jennifer's beauty routine must be streamlined, since she has little time to herself. She wants a fresh and natural, healthy and youthful daytime look. With a tight schedule in which care of her family is the top priority, she likes to save time on beauty care without cutting important corners.

Since her **skin** is oily, Jennifer has to cleanse it in the morning as well as at night. She uses her mask every other day as part of her evening cleansing routine to keep oiliness under control. After her regular cleansing and masking, Jennifer uses a protecting liquid foundation to help reduce shine on her facial skin. She then applies basic daytime **makeup**: translucent face powder in a light peach shade; brown eyebrow pencil to match her coloring; a medium plum eye shadow on her lids with a pale, pearly pink highlighter on the browbone; a brown eyeliner and mascara; and a soft coral lip color. Jennifer's morning skin-care and makeup routine takes a total of fifteen minutes and gives her a fresh, soft look all day — with just a few touch-ups of lip color. For evenings out, Jennifer adds a darker plum eye shadow for contour, applies a contour blusher shade under her daytime blusher, and a brighter coral tone to her lips.

Jennifer wears her **hair** shoulder length because she likes the versatility of wearing it down at night and up and away from her face during the day. Because her hair tends to be oily she washes it every day, conditioning just the ends to prevent tangling. Jennifer's hair is thickly distributed, fine in texture, and very straight — an ideal combination for shoulder-length hair — and she allows it to dry naturally after washing. Before evenings out, Jennifer uses an intensive conditioner on the bottom half of hair shafts to protect them and make them extra shiny. After it dries she puts her hair in electric rollers to add elegant volume with curls.

Jennifer's two calisthenics classes a week help keep her **body** toned, and for fun and relaxation she plays tennis with a friend at least once a week for ninety minutes. Her choice of fragrances suits her romantic personality and is based on floral notes. For daytime she likes to express a joyful mood with green fragrances; for evenings out she likes the elegance of chypres. The basis of Jennifer's

Jennifer's busy schedule demands a beauty routine that's efficient and effective. Her morning regimen takes just fifteen minutes, and she's ready for the day's many activities.

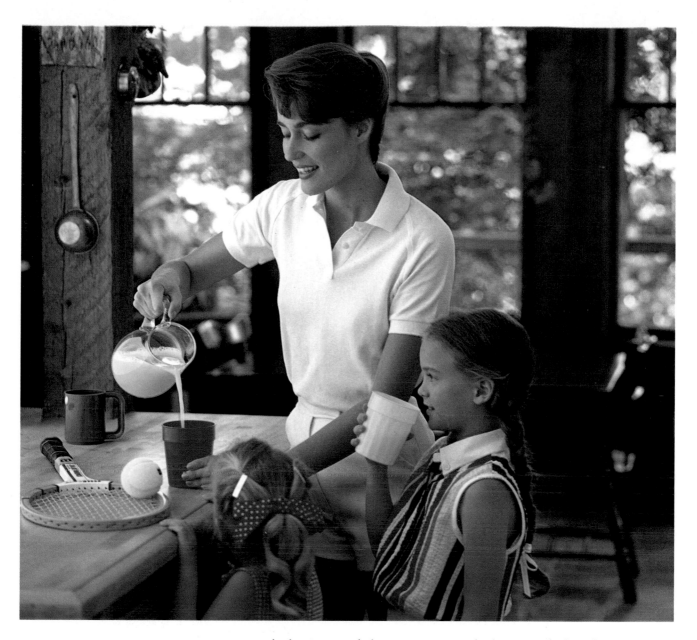

wardrobe is casual daytime wear, with dressier clothes for evening. Turtleneck tops and sweaters help make her neck appear shorter, and skirts with gathered waistlines, hemmed at mid-knee, add desired shape to her bottom while diminishing her height. For evening, Jennifer chooses a romantic style: high-necked, ruffled blouses or dresses and full skirts with a great deal of detail at her waist.

Beauty musts: keeping skin and hair clean to control oiliness; using versatile makeup and hair-styling techniques for quick day-to-evening transitions; protecting her skin with sunscreen when she's out of doors, especially playing tennis; and at least once a week, an evening beauty bath after a hectic day.

Putting It All Together

Carol, a career woman on the go, needs a beauty routine that's well organized. To achieve the professional look she needs every day, her morning beauty routine emphasizes glamour makeup.

Carol is a single career woman who travels frequently. She needs time in the morning to put together a sophisticated business look, so she adjusts her beauty routine with trade-offs — a short, simple hairstyle gives Carol more time for makeup, and a superorganized wardrobe helps her make efficient choices when she's in a hurry.

Carol's dry *skin* needs extra protection because she spends so much time in the dehydrating atmosphere of airplanes. She moisturizes daily and always uses sunscreen, knowing she will be outdoors at least part of every day. After applying a creamy, protective foundation, Carol begins her *makeup* routine with translucent face powder and a cream cheek color to accent her cheekbones, then applies a soft berry tone blusher. For sophisticated daytime eyes,

Carol uses deep green and cocoa eye shadow with a slate eye-defining pencil. For lip color, she uses a lip pencil in a pink tone, filling in with a bright rose, then adds lots of gloss. For evenings out, she touches up her blusher by using a more intense tone over her daytime shade, and adds a shell eye shadow to her inner eyelid. She gives her evening lips extra dimension by first lining them, then using a darker rose shade.

Carol keeps her naturally blond *hair* short in a soft style that flatters her oval face. She brightens the color of her dry hair with professional highlighting, so she needs a regular conditioner every time she washes her hair and an intensive conditioner after every other shampoo. The conditioners help hold moisture and shine in Carol's hair when she styles it with a blow-dryer after washings. She uses decorated combs to pull one side of her hair back for dressy evenings.

Carol takes extra care to apply moisturizer all over her *body* every day. She also finds regular aerobic exercise essential to developing the stamina she needs every day. Jogging thirty minutes at least three times a week is ideal for her lifestyle, since she can do it anywhere, even when she travels. She also swims as often as she can. Carol favors spicy scents that convey her adventurous personality: for daytime she wears the fresh scent of green fragrances; for evening she prefers the mysterious mood created by Oriental fragrance notes. To give needed volume to her upper body and bustline, Carol's daytime business fashion is full-shaped blouses in light, bright colors and slimmer-cut skirts, nipped at the waist. She keeps her skirt lengths at mid-knee and jackets just below her waist to give her legs a more elongated look. For evening Carol finds that puffy sleeves and narrow skirts worn with bright belts and high-heeled sandals add dimension to her bustline and length to her legs.

Beauty musts: moisturizing and protecting her dry skin to keep it fresh and dewy; simple hair styling that allows plenty of time for morning makeup; regular aerobic exercise for added energy; and layering fragrance to make it last.

Putting It All Together

Gail is a working mother who runs a consulting business from her home. She works from early morning until midafternoon, when her children come home from grade school. Since her life is varied and busy, with many professional and household responsibilities, Gail schedules different elements of her beauty routine throughout the day.

Gail's **skin** is normal in type and light in tone, so she puts effort into maintaining its condition with regular skin care that emphasizes sunscreen protection. Since Gail's time with her children is often spent outdoors, she uses a sunscreen under her makeup every day. Her **makeup** needs vary from a natural, easy look for home, to the professional polish she needs for business appointments, to a dressier appearance for evenings out. After freshening her skin and protecting it (with sunscreen and foundation) in the morning, Gail uses the Glamour Basics daytime look to start the day. Before business appointments she adds the sophistication of contouring effects with a pink blusher to give more definite angles to her cheeks and reduce their width; Gail blends highlighter into her foundation at the top of her cheekbones, strokes blusher on under the highlighter and a contour blusher under the lighter shade, blending it to her hairline. For a sophisticated daytime eye look, she brings her basic blue lid color down under her eye to the lower lash base and adds a deeper green for contour in the crease, between the blue lid shade and a shell highlighter on the brow-bone. To make her eyes appear larger, she extends the medium blue lid color slightly beyond the outer corner of her eyes and outlines top and bottom lids with a blue eye-defining pencil. She outlines her lips with a deep-toned lip pencil, filling in with a crimson lip color, then whisks on a glimmer of gloss.

For her evening look, Gail uses the same basic techniques that work for her business look but brightens the colors.

Gail wears her **hair** medium length, allowing her to style it in a way that is most flattering to her square jawline. She sometimes pulls her hair back at her ears with combs, a style ideal for both

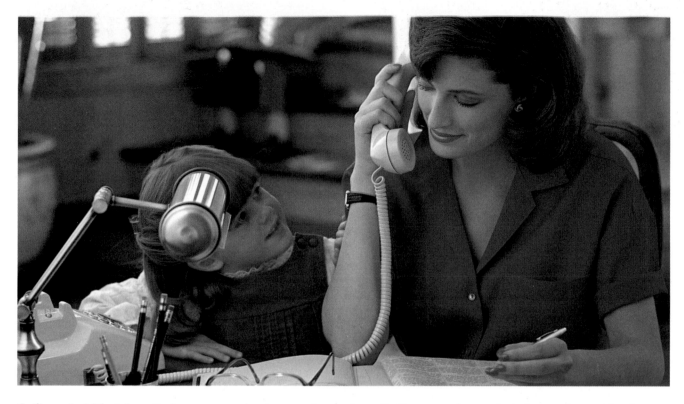

Gail's varied lifestyle calls for a beauty routine that's very versatile. By adapting her basic glamour makeup, she's able to achieve a range of looks to suit her many needs.

daytime and evening. Gail's normal-type hair has to be washed every two or three days. She always uses a conditioner to prevent tangling after shampooing; after every fourth shampoo, she uses an intensive conditioner for extra body and bounce.

To keep her *body* fit, Gail finds that she can work regular aerobic exercise into the afternoons she spends with her children by going bicycle riding with them. For relaxing stretches she attends an evening yoga class once or twice a week. The fragrances Gail favors express her sophisticated personality: for day she likes the softness of floral fragrances and for evening she prefers the gracious aura of aldehydics. She also has a wardrobe of fragrances to suit different occasions — herbaceous scents for sporty family outings, more sophisticated Orientals for daytime career meetings, and chypres for romantic evenings. Gail dresses her full figure for business days in clean, elongated lines in suit jackets, keeping her color scheme to dark, subtle hues. For evening she favors simple, elegant black, accented with dramatic accessories and large-scale jewelry. She looks for extended shoulders in many of her shirts and jackets to balance her full hips and legs, and wears long, straight-shaped skirts for dressy evenings.

Beauty musts: consistent skin and hair care emphasizing protection to maintain their normal condition; using contrasting colors to change her makeup look from day to evening; keeping wardrobe colors well coordinated, simple, and flattering; having a variety of fragrances to suit all her moods and occasions.

Total Beauty

The glow of total beauty radiates from within.
It is the glorious culmination of all that is
beautiful about you — your personality, your
skin, your makeup, your hair, and your body.
Only you hold the key to total beauty — only
you can make the difference!

Making It Yours

You're a beautiful woman — you've worked hard at developing your own inner beauty, and we hope that all you've learned on the previous pages has helped to bring your own special beauty to the surface.

Your thoughtful answers to all the inventory questions throughout this book — especially on the following two pages — demonstrate your interest in every aspect of yourself. And because interest, caring, and commitment are the most important requirements for obtaining the best results from a complete beauty program, the effort, enthusiasm, and self-knowledge you invest in the guidelines you've learned will help make the difference.

But only you make the real difference — your time and effort, your special attention to details and problems, your caring about who you are and how you look. Making all of it yours — your inner beauty, your skin care, your glamorous makeup, your hair care, and your overall body care — means giving priority to your own health and beauty because you know how important they are to the way you feel about yourself and about the world around you. And you want to present your personal best, the most beautiful you possible, *every day* to *everyone*.

2 *Skin Care*
The basis of becoming and being your beautiful best; giving your skin the care and attention it needs by following the five steps to beautiful skin — cleanse, **retexture**, freshen, moisture balance, and protect; paying attention to the importance of your skin's health and appearance by really working at — and *enjoying* — the time and effort you devote to giving your skin a radiant glow, a smooth, even surface you can see, a soft, dewy texture you can feel: the perfect reflection of the very special way you've learned to care for yourself.

1 *Your Special Beauty*
Your understanding of who you are and your appreciation of your best inner qualities, wisely combined with those areas of your character you're always working on, always making better.

3 *Glamour Makeup*

The techniques and colors you choose to enhance your features — your eyes, lips, cheeks; the way you use the most sophisticated beauty knowledge to add a soft, natural glow to your face or to dramatize your looks with special effects; being adventurous and experimenting with makeup, learning new ways to look that you may never have thought were possible for you, understanding the nature of makeup and how to use it to your most beautiful advantage.

4 *Hair Care*

The special care you take to make the most of your hair's natural beauty: keeping it clean, soft, and conditioned, alive with shine and vitality, silky and lustrous, styled to enhance its natural characteristics and to frame your face beautifully.

5 *Body Care*

The total image you project by putting it all together beautifully, paying attention to all the details — your hands, your feet, the sleep you get, and your fragrance choices and wardrobe — making them all part of a complete beauty routine that works for you, giving your body skin the extra care it needs to look soft and toned, to feel youthfully silken, and to retain its special beauty.

Taking a Final Look

Now that you have read *The Mary Kay Guide to Beauty*, take time to complete a few more statements and evaluate your overall appearance and feelings. Answer thoughtfully and honestly, and use your answers to help you set new goals for becoming all you can be.

This inventory includes a reference source of page numbers to give you extra instruction and inspiration in the specific areas covered in this book.

1. **I would like to increase my potential for inner beauty by concentrating more on the following areas:**
   □ Self-confidence (*see pages 20 and 21*)
   □ Intimacy (*see pages 22 and 23*)
   □ Inner strength (*see pages 24 and 25*)
   □ Versatility (*see pages 26 and 27*)
   □ Direction (*see pages 28 and 29*)
   □ Self-fulfillment (*see pages 30 and 31*)
   □ Positive attitude (*see pages 32 and 33*)

2. **I understand the structure and composition of skin and the scientific basis for skin care.**
   □ Yes
   □ No (*see pages 40 to 43*)

3. **I would like my skin to look and feel (check all that apply):**
   □ Clearer, with fewer clogged pores and breakouts (*see pages 56 to 59*)
   □ Brighter and more translucent (*see pages 60 and 61*)
   □ Fresher and better toned (*see pages 62 and 63*)
   □ Softer, smoother, less dry, and better conditioned (*see pages 64 to 67*)
   □ More youthful, more even toned in texture, and less wrinkled (*see pages 68 to 73*)

4. **I use a sunscreen to prevent sun damage on my facial skin:**
   □ Whenever I will be outdoors, regardless of the season or the weather
   □ Only when I know I will be directly exposed to the sun (*see pages 46, 47, and 73*)
   □ Occasionally: when I go to the beach or boating (*see pages 46, 47, and 73*)
   □ Infrequently: I like to get a tan (*see pages 46, 47, and 73*)

5. **I feel the time I currently spend on skin care is:**
   □ Steadily improving the way my skin looks and feels
   □ Not producing the results I'd like to see in my skin (*see pages 54 to 73*)

6. **I am happy with my total daytime makeup look:**
   □ Always, or most of the time
   □ Sometimes, but I need to learn new techniques (*see pages 80 to 115*)

7. **My makeup remains in good condition until I've used it up.**
   □ Yes
   □ No (*see page 81*)

8. **I would like my face to appear (check either or both):**
   □ More contoured and structured, with highlights (*see page 97*)
   □ Less blotchy and irregular in coloring, with fewer obvious blemishes, lines, and dark areas (*see page 97*)

9. **I need to improve my application of daytime (check all that apply):**
   □ Cheek color (*see pages 92 to 95*)
   □ Eyebrow pencil (*see pages 100 and 101*)
   □ Eye shadow (*see pages 102 to 105*)
   □ Eyeliner and/or eye-defining pencil (*see pages 106 and 107*)
   □ Mascara (*see pages 108 and 109*)
   □ Lip color (*see pages 112 and 113*)

10. **For specific effects, I would like to learn how to experiment more with (check all that apply):**
    □ My makeup colors (*see pages 82 to 91*)
    □ Cheek contouring (*see pages 98 to 99*)
    □ Enhancing the size, shape, and/ or setting of my eyes (*see pages 110 and 111*)
    □ Flattering eyeglass shapes (*see page 99*)
    □ Enhancing the size and/or shape of my lips (*see pages 114 and 115*)

11. I understand the structure and composition of hair and the scientific basis for hair care.
    □ Yes
    □ No (*see pages 148 and 149*)

12. I would like my hair to look and feel (check all that apply):
    □ Cleaner and fresher (*see pages 154 and 155*)
    □ More flexible, shinier, less fly-away (*see pages 156 and 157*)
    □ Less damaged, with fewer split and broken ends (*see pages 158 and 159*)

13. I am concerned about (check all that apply):
    □ Dandruff (*see page 160*)
    □ Dry scalp (*see page 160*)
    □ Hair loss (*see pages 160 and 161*)
    □ How coloring and other treatments affect my hair (*see pages 162 and 163*)

14. I need new hair styling ideas for (check all that apply):
    □ Finding a hairstyle that suits the characteristic of my hair (*see pages 164 and 165*)
    □ Styling my hair to flatter my face (*see pages 166 to 169*)
    □ Adding versatility and special effects to my hairstyle (*see page 167*)

15. I feel the time I currently spend on hair care is:
    □ Steadily improving the way my hair looks and feels
    □ Not producing the results I'd like to see in my hair (*see pages 150 to 169*)

16. I understand the structure and composition of body skin and the scientific basis for body skin care.
    □ Yes
    □ No (*see pages 178 to 181*)

17. I would like my body skin to look and feel (check all that apply):
    □ Cleaner, fresher, and softer (*see pages 188 and 189*)
    □ Smoother; more polished looking; less rough on elbows, feet, and knees (*see pages 190 and 191*)
    □ Silkier, less dry (*see pages 192 and 193*)

18. I use sunscreen on my body skin:
    □ Whenever I am outdoors, regardless of the season or the weather
    □ Only when I know I will be directly exposed to the sun (*see pages 46, 47, 194, and 195*)
    □ Occasionally: when I go to the beach or boating (*see pages 46, 47, and 195*)
    □ Infrequently: I like to get a tan (*see pages 46, 47, and 195*)

19. I need more information on the following areas of concern regarding body care (check all that apply):
    □ My hands (*see pages 196 to 199*)
    □ My feet (*see pages 200 and 201*)

□ Hair removal (*see pages 202 and 203*)
□ During my pregnancy (*see pages 204 and 205*)
□ Nutrition and vitamins (*see pages 206 to 209*)
□ Exercise (*see pages 210 and 211*)
□ Sleep and relaxation (*see pages 212 to 213*)

20. I'd like to learn new ideas about (check all that apply):
    □ Fragrances that suit my individual personality, mood, and preferences (*see pages 216 and 217*)
    □ Buying the right fragrance for myself (*see pages 218 and 219*)
    □ Wearing fragrance in different ways (*see pages 218 and 219*)
    □ Using fragrance in layers (*see page 220*)

21. Rank the following elements of your total beauty routine from one to five, beginning with the element that gives you the best results. Then reread the sections on those elements you feel still need some work.
    □ Skin care (*see pages 38 to 75*)
    □ Daytime makeup (*see pages 76 to 117*)
    □ Special makeup effects (*see pages 118 to 145*)
    □ Hair care (*see pages 146 to 175*)
    □ Body care (*see pages 176 to 195*)
    □ Nutrition (*see pages 206 to 209*)

You Make the Difference!

The dawn of a new you: making the most of who you are, understanding and expressing your own style of beauty, which begins inside you and emerges to tell others what a special person you are.

Your beauty begins with a healthy, radiant complexion that comes only from understanding your skin and your commitment to a daily skin-care routine. It stems from your knowledgeable use of glamour makeup — your ability to achieve just the right look for every occasion, experimenting with what you've learned, being adventurous, and taking your own glamorous look to the limit. Total beauty also includes proper hair care — keeping it clean, conditioned, styled, and feeling as lovely as it looks. And next, body care: paying attention to every inch of skin on your body. Finally, beauty means paying attention to important details, developing your fragrance and fashion senses.

Your personal beauty begins here — with the dawn of the new you who knows how to do it right, put it all together, and make it yours — beautifully yours — starting now!

Glossary

Acid balance — the natural pH level of the skin's surface moisture: *see* pH

Aerobic exercise — activity that increases lung activity so that greater amounts of oxygen are absorbed and the heart rate is increased

Aldehydics — one of five general fragrance categories

Alkali — any of various water-soluble mineral salts with a pH greater than 7; a quality of detergent soaps

Allergen — a substance that produces an allergic reaction

Allergy — a hypersensitive reaction

Alopecia areata — a scalp disorder resulting in bald patches, believed to be related to "autoimmunity," or the body becoming allergic to its own chemicals

Androgen — a class of hormones that includes the male hormone testosterone; also a component of some birth-control pills

Apocrine sweat glands — small tubes that secrete a milky substance that develops the characteristic human odor as it is decomposed by bacteria on the skin's surface; found mainly in the underarms, around the nipples, and in the groin

Arrector pili muscle — a muscle attached to each hair follicle that contracts as a result of cold or fear, making the hair shaft stand up straight and produce "goose bumps"

Astringent — causing the drawing together or constricting of tissue, such as skin or scalp; causing

pores to appear smaller; may also refer to a lotion that produces such action

Atopic dermatitis (*see* eczema) —

Bacteria — one-celled organisms of various kinds, some of which cause infection

Birthmark — dark areas of the skin produced by excessive pigmentation

Blood vessels — vessels that supply nutrients and oxygen to the skin; they help regulate body temperature by contracting and expanding in response to external stimuli

Browbone — the usually prominent area just under the outer half of the eyebrow; a ridgelike bone found under the length of the eyebrow

Callus — hard, tough skin, created by friction

Capillaries — minute blood vessels that connect arteries and veins

Chloasma — "mask of pregnancy," dark patches on cheeks, near mouth or brow, associated with hormonal changes of pregnancy

Chypres — one of five general fragrance categories

Collagen — a protein substance found in connective or supportive tissue such as the dermis

Color family — a group of colors with the same undertone — warm (yellow) or cool (blue)

Color harmony — a look that is achieved by using cheek colors and lip colors from the same color family — both warm or both cool

Comedo — technical name for skin

lesions, which include blackheads (open comedones) and whiteheads (closed comedones)

Comedogenic — causing comedones — whiteheads or blackheads

Contouring (as related to makeup) — adding dimension with shadows and highlights to any of the facial features

Cool colors — colors with blue undertones

Cortex (hair) — the middle layer of the hair surrounded by the cuticle (the outermost layer) and protecting the innermost layer, the medulla

Cosmetic — a beautifying agent, usually for the face or body

Cuticle (hair) — the thin, hard outer surface of the hair shaft; covers the cortex

Cuticle (nails) — the hard skin at the base and sides of fingernails and toenails

Definition (as related to makeup) — emphasis or accent on the shape or contour of any of the facial features

Dehydration — the loss or absence of moisture or water

Demarcation (in makeup application) — the obvious boundary line between two shades or textures; the unappealing effect of makeup that is not well blended and/or shows an unattractive line between skin and makeup

Depilatory — a chemical compound for removing hair

Dermatology — the medical study and science of the structure, function, and diseases of the skin

Dermis — the fibrous skin layer beneath the epidermis, composed primarily of elastin and collagen

Detergent — a product designed to clean hair and skin from substances such as oils, environmental pollutants, etc.

DNA — *d*eoxyribo*n*ucleic *a*cid. a complex chromosomal component of the nuclei, or centers, of living cells, which determine individual hereditary characteristics

Dormancy — a period of rest, when growth ceases (in hair, for example)

Eccrine sweat glands — small coiled tubes that open up on the skin's surface as pores, bringing water and waste products (perspiration) to the skin's surface

Eczema — a wide range of skin problems, usually related to an extreme susceptibility to some form of irritation or allergy

Elasticity — the capacity (as of skin or hair) to stretch without losing shape

Elastin — a substance that forms a principal component of elastic fiber or tissue in the body, found in the dermis layer; it keeps the skin supple

Emery board — a cardboard nail-filing implement coated with a fine-grained aluminum oxide or other abrasive mineral; used to grind and polish the nail gently

Emollient — a substance that softens and soothes, usually by depositing oil on the skin's surface

Epidermis — the outermost layer of skin cells covering the body; the skin we can see

Fibrocytes — cells that produce high-tensile-strength fibers made of the protein collagen, the "structural steel" of the skin

Hair follicles — tubes in which hair grows; they originate in the dermis and extend upward through the epidermis, forming the surrounding tissue for growing hair

Heredity — the genetic transmission of characteristics from parents to offspring

Hormones — substances produced by several of the body's organs that stimulate other organs to function by chemical activity

Horny layer (*see stratum corneum*) —

Hue — the designation of the color itself, such as red, blue, yellow, etc.

Humectants — water-attracting, or moisture-binding, substances

Humidity — the amount of moisture or water held in the atmosphere

Hydrate — to moisturize or add water

Hyperactivity — a high level of activity in the functioning of organs or glands (such as sebaceous glands)

Intensity — the degree of saturation or concentration in a color — or its brightness or dullness; more intense hues are vivid (a heavy concentration of color), less intense hues are soft (a light concentration of color)

Iris (of the eye) — the colored circular area surrounding the eye's pupil

Irritant — any condition or substance that produces irritation

Keratin — a tough, fibrous protein that is part of the outer layer of the skin's epidermis and of the hair and fingernails

Lubrication — the coating on a material or skin which promotes mobility and reduces friction

Manicure stick — a nail-care implement made of soft wood (like orange), usually with a pointed end for cleaning and a flat, round end for grooming the nail cuticle

Matte finish — an even-toned, non-shiny surface quality (as of skin to which translucent powder has been applied)

Medulla (hair) — the innermost, softest substance that forms the center of some hair shafts

Melanin — A dark skin and hair pigment

Melanocytes — cells producing melanin

Mid-shaft split — the unraveling of the ropelike fibers of the cortex in the middle of a shaft of hair

Natural bristle brush — a brush made from natural animal hair (often boar) rather than synthetics such as plastic; generally considered to be gentler on the hair and scalp

Neutral colors — colors that have neither yellow nor blue undertones, such as gray; in working with glamour makeup, shades that contain a very small amount of color and/or those that harmonize with either warm or cool colors may also be referred to as neutrals

Glossary

Opaque — not allowing light to penetrate — the opposite of transparent; dense coverage

Oxidation — simply put, the combination of any substance with oxygen

Papule — a small, inflamed elevation of the skin

Patina — a fine, smooth film, usually glowing, that forms on a surface

pH (*potential of Hydrogen*) — a measure of acidity or alkalinity of a solution or substance; 7 is neutral pH; lower pH numbers represent acid pH, high pH numbers indicate alkaline pH; the natural pH of skin is slightly acidic, or below pH 7

Pigment — any coloring agent, such as melanin, in the skin and hair

Pollutant — impure or unclean contaminating materials

Psoriasis — a skin condition characterized by patches of scaly, shedding skin; most often develops on the scalp, knees, and elbows

Pumice — a porous, lightweight, abrasive volcanic stone used to soften and polish hard, tough, or callused skin

Regenerate — re-create living material, or renew functioning

Rosacea — a face rash that produces redness and pimples in adults, especially on the nose, mid-forehead, chin, and cheeks

Saturated color — dense, opaque makeup colors, applied so that little of the natural skin tones show through

Scar — connective tissue visible at the skin's surface that fills in the opening of a cut

Sebaceous glands — oil-producing glands attached to hair follicles

Seborrheic dermatitis — a common skin disorder that produces scaling and itching of the facial skin; may be associated with excessive secretion of sebum

Sebum — a semiliquid oil secreted by the sebaceous glands that lubricates the skin's surface

Shafts (of hair) — individual strands of hair

Sloughing — the shedding of an outer layer of dead tissue from a living structure, such as skin

SPF (Sun Protection Factor) — the numerical rating on sunscreens that indicates the level of protection they can provide the skin from ultraviolet radiation; the higher the SPF number, the greater a sunscreen's protective capacity

Split end — the unraveling of the ropelike fibers of the cortex at the end of a shaft of hair

Stratum corneum — the flat, dead skin cells that form a protective outer layer on the surface of the skin; also called horny layer

Subcutaneous — below the skin

Sunscreen — a preparation that, depending on its SPF factor, absorbs in varying degrees the harmful burning rays of the sun

Translucent — allowing some light to penetrate or pass through, without being completely transparent

T-zone — the T-shaped area of the face formed by the forehead, the nose, and the chin, which sometimes tends to be oilier than other facial areas

Ultraviolet — the range of light wavelengths (usually from the sun) between violet radiation in the visible spectrum and the invisible x-ray spectrum; such rays are harmful to the skin

Value — the amount of lightness or darkness in a color, achieved by adding white or black

Vitiligo — light patches on the skin resulting from the lack of melanin in a specific area

Warm colors — colors with yellow, or golden, undertones

Water-resistant — repelling moisture or water; not easily rinsed away by water

Water-soluble — the quality of dissolving in water; easily removed with water

Mary Kay Cosmetics, Inc., fully supports skin-care education and research through: Harvard University–the Massachusetts Institute of Technology, Division of Health Sciences and Technology; the University of Texas Health Science Center at Dallas; and the "Skin Deep" exhibit, developed by Mary Kay Cosmetics, Inc., in cooperation with the American Academy of Dermatology, the Dermatology Foundation, the Chicago Dermatology Society, and the Museum of Science and Industry in Chicago, Illinois.

Index

All photographs in *The Mary Kay Guide to Beauty* are the work of Tim Boole, Steve Seeger, and Neill Whitlock with the exception of the following: 7, Francesco Scavullo; 13 and 25, Ilse Thoma/The Image Bank; 14 (top) and 56, Hank Londoner/The Image Bank; 14 (bottom) and 46 (bottom), Miguel/The Image Bank; 15, Nancy Brown/The Image Bank; 16 (top), 29, 32, 33, 34 (top), 42, and 212, Skip Hine; 16 (bottom), D. Kugelmeier/The Image Bank; 17, John Stember/The Image Bank; 18, Philip M. Prosen/The Image Bank; 19 (top), Whitney Lane/The Image Bank; 19 (bottom), Richard Steedman/The Image Bank; 20, Elisabeth Weiland/Photo Researchers; 21 (top), Steve Niedorf/The Image Bank; 21 (bottom) and 205, Elyse Lewin/The Image Bank; 22, Werner Bokelberg/The Image Bank; 23, George Hausman/The Image Bank; 24, Jay Maisel/The Image Bank; 26, Paulo Rocha/The Image Bank; 27, Alvis Upitis/The Image Bank; 28, Steve Dunnell/The Image Bank; 30, Edward Leptau/Photo Researchers; 31, Faustino R/The Image Bank; 35, Jack Ward/The Image Bank; 43 (right), 185, and 213, Larry Dale Gordon/The Image Bank; 45, Rosemary Howard; 46 (top), Susan McCartney/Photo Researchers; 73, Jean Louis Sauverzac/The Image Bank; 78, Janeart, LTD/The Image Bank; 79 (left), Gabe Palmer/The Image Bank; 79 (right), Brett H. Froomer/The Image Bank; 109 (lower right), Michael Salas/The Image Bank; 195 (top), John Kelly/The Image Bank; 195 (bottom), David Brownell/The Image Bank.